W0234936

Ethics and the Good Nurse

Ethics and the Good Nurse draws on internationally leading empirical research conducted by the Jubilee Centre for Character and Virtues and explores nursing as a virtuous profession through a close examination of nurses' character.

With the belief that virtues such as kindness, integrity, compassion and honesty are core to the nursing profession, this book draws on extended insights from the Jubilee Centre's *Virtuous Practicing in Nursing* study to understand the role of such virtues in the professional practice and education of nurses. This book brings together knowledge from academics, scholars and practitioners to address the influence of personal and professional character on nurses and nursing.

By including clear implications for policy, practice and research, *Ethics and the Good Nurse* serves as essential reading for a wide audience, including nurses, policy makers and nursing organisations and provides a timely and much-needed contribution to the field of nursing and character education.

Andrew Peterson is Professor of Character and Citizenship Education and Deputy Director of the Jubilee Centre for Character and Virtues at the University of Birmingham, UK.

James Arthur is Professor of Education and Civic Engagement and Director of the Jubilee Centre for Character and Virtues at the University of Birmingham, UK.

Jinu Varghese is a lecturer at the School of Nursing, University of Birmingham, UK.

Character and Virtue within the Professions

Series Editors

James Arthur, *Professor of Education and Civic Engagement and Director of the Jubilee Centre for Character and Virtues at the University of Birmingham, UK.*

Andrew Peterson, *Professor of Character and Citizenship Education and Deputy Director of the Jubilee Centre for Character and Virtues at the University of Birmingham, UK.*

The principal objective of the series is to highlight the interplay between practitioners' personal character and the ethical dimensions of their professional domain. Each book will explore the specific ethical dimensions of the given profession at hand, including the interplay between professionals' individual character virtues and their working environments. In a time when cultures of managerialism, auditing, performance metrics and commercial success are seemingly increasing, this series attempts to re-focus the professions towards the ethical and societal origins that each profession intends to serve. Underpinned by perspectives of philosophy, psychology and sociology, each book will offer practitioners fresh viewpoints about how their character and professional context can influence their professional practice.

Books in the series include:

Ethics and the Good Teacher
Character in the Professional Domain
Andrew Peterson with James Arthur

Ethics and the Good Doctor
Character in the Professional Domain
Dr. Sabena Jameel, Andrew Peterson and James Arthur

Ethics and the Good Nurse
Character in the Professional Domain
Andrew Peterson, James Arthur and Jinu Varghese

For more information about this series, please visit: www.routledge.com/Character-and-Virtue-Within-the-Professions/book-series/CVP

Ethics and the Good Nurse

Character in the Professional Domain

Andrew Peterson, James Arthur and Jinu Varghese

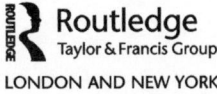

Routledge
Taylor & Francis Group

LONDON AND NEW YORK

First published 2022
by Routledge
2 Park Square, Milton Park, Abingdon, Oxon OX14 4RN

and by Routledge
605 Third Avenue, New York, NY 10158

Routledge is an imprint of the Taylor & Francis Group, an informa business

© 2022 Andrew Peterson, James Arthur, and Jinu Varghese

The right of Andrew Peterson, James Arthur, and Jinu Varghese to be identified as authors of this work has been asserted in accordance with sections 77 and 78 of the Copyright, Designs and Patents Act 1988.

British Library Cataloguing-in-Publication Data
A catalogue record for this book is available from the British Library

Library of Congress Cataloging-in-Publication Data
A catalog record for this book has been requested

ISBN: 978-0-367-70432-2 (hbk)
ISBN: 978-0-367-70434-6 (pbk)
ISBN: 978-1-003-14630-8 (ebk)

DOI: 10.4324/9781003146308

Typeset in Times New Roman
by Apex CoVantage, LLC

Contents

Acknowledgements

This book is the third in a series of texts that examine *Character and Virtues in the Professions*. Each book in the series is dedicated to a specific profession and brings together reviews of existing literature and sources of empirical data – including data collected in various projects by the Jubilee Centre for Character and Virtues – to provide new insights for both pre- and in-service professionals, as well as acting as an educational resource to inform future professional decision-making and practice.

As we make clear from the outset, this book draws extensively on data and analysis from one of a number of research projects on virtues in the professions conducted and reported on by the Jubilee Centre that were all led by the Centre's Director, James Arthur. For this reason, we owe our sincere gratitude to those colleagues whose data collection, analysis, recommendations and overall insight on the project reported here including in the resulting report have made this book possible. In particular, our thanks and acknowledgements go to Kristján Kristjánsson and Francisco Moller. We are also grateful to our colleagues at Routledge – in particular Anna Clarkson, Sarah Hyde, Will Bateman and Akshara Dafre – for their interest and support in this series and book.

Andrew Peterson
James Arthur
Jinu Varghese

Introduction

Introduction

This book, and the main study from which the data contained within it are drawn, are based on the conviction that being a 'good' nurse is an inherently moral activity. While being a good nurse does involve possessing requisite medical knowledge and the ability to apply that knowledge appropriately and effectively, as is widely known and believed 'good' nursing requires compassion, care, empathy and a range of other related dispositions – or as we refer to them in this book, virtues. These virtues lie at the heart of the nursing profession and feature heavily in official documents and in patient testimonies regarding what they desire from nurses who treat them. For example, the Nursing and Midwifery Council's[1] (NMC, 2020: 6) code of professional standards of practice and behaviour emphasises the need to 'prioritise people', to 'treat people as individuals and uphold their dignity' and to 'treat people with kindness, respect and compassion'. As with other professions, a core constituent of the relationship between nurses and their patients is trust, and the Code emphasises that trust is promoted through professionalism. This trust is essential given that nursing is fundamentally concerned with the care of vulnerable human beings (Titchen, 2000).

Recognising that nursing involves an ethical dimension and requires the development and practice of certain dispositions is one thing, but precisely framing and detailing the contours and depth of these is another. As we consider and explore in the chapters of this book, there has been significant attention to the ethical nature of nursing within academic literature and public policy over at least the last two decades. As we also examine, a notable feature of this attention has been the extent to which various factors – including changes to healthcare systems, the cultures of settings (healthcare trusts, hospitals and so on) and nursing education – act to either (or both) support and constrain the moral nature of nursing. In this regard, the nursing profession is not unique, with broadly comparable interest also

DOI: 10.4324/9781003146308-1

evident in the moral dimensions of a number of professions. Similarly, as once again is commonly cited within the extant literature examined in Chapters 1 and 2 of this book, over the last few decades, nursing practice has become heavily impacted by the processes of marketisation and regulatory accountability that shape healthcare systems in many countries today. Though these processes are not necessarily and always inimical to ethical practice, the pressures of external targets, working conditions, competition between providers and pressure on resources all affect how nurses care for their patients.

Since its inception in 2012, the Jubilee Centre for Character and Virtues based at the University of Birmingham has conducted numerous studies that have sought the views, perceptions and explanations of professionals themselves in order to interrogate and explore the ethical dimensions of professions in England, each led by the Centre's Director, Professor James Arthur. In this book, we draw on data from one of these studies – *Virtuous Practice in Nursing* – to present and analyse how nurses at three stages of their careers – (first year) Undergraduate Students, Graduating Students and Experienced Nurses (we explain each of these categories in the following section) – understand the ethical dimensions of their work. While we add some additional analysis to the findings, including reporting additional qualitative data from the study and entering into conversation with relevant research literature published since the study, this book draws extensively the original research report produced by the project (Kristjánsson, Varghese *et al.*, 2017). Our intention is to bring this study to a new audience and to draw deeper connections with existing literature in the field of nursing ethics and virtue. In addition, in this book, we draw more extensively on the interview data gathered than was possible in the space of the original report.

The Centre's work on the ethical dimensions of nursing as a profession has also been detailed in various articles and books published by the Centre members on nursing itself (see, e.g., Varghese and Kristjánsson, 2018) and on the professions more widely (e.g., Arthur *et al.*, 2014; Arthur, Kristjánsson, Thomas *et al.*, 2015; Arthur, Kristjánsson, Cooke *et al.*, 2015; Arthur *et al.*, 2018, 2019a; Harrison and Khatoon, 2017; Kristjánsson, 2015a; Kristjánsson *et al.*, 2017a).

Our aim in this introductory chapter is twofold. First, we provide summary details of the main project drawn upon in our analysis. For reasons of space and concision, we present a summary of the main aims, research questions and methods for each of these projects. The detailed aims, research questions and methods of each of this project can be found on the Jubilee Centre's website.[2] Second, we set out the structure of the book, including the focus and broad content of each of the chapters that follow.

The project

The *Virtuous Practice in Nursing* project was a two-year study, in Great Britain, involving first-year undergraduate nursing students (referred to throughout as *First-Year Undergraduate Students*), students who had recently graduated from their course (referred to throughout as *Final-Year Undergraduate Students*) and nurses with at least five years of experience (referred to throughout as *Experienced Nurses*). The study also sought the views of educators from the UK schools of nursing. The overarching aim of the *Virtuous Practice in Nursing* project was to identify which personal virtues nursing students and experienced nurses understood themselves as holding and to investigate how these were viewed as influencing their professional lives. A central concern of the study, given the extant literature (examined in Chapters 1 and 2) and the Jubilee Centre for Character and Virtues' interest in professional character, was to explore the extent to which nurses relied – and were required to rely – upon codes of practice and guidelines in making decisions and how these interacted with their own beliefs and conceptions of professional virtues. Recognising that professionals work within institutional, regulatory and disciplinary frameworks, which are meant to serve a 'public-protection' function, the project explored how these restrict and/or allow space for individual moral agency.

The main research questions that guided the project were as follows:

1 Which virtues are prized and upheld by nursing students and nurses, according to self-reports?
2 Which virtues do they associate with the 'ideal' professional?
3 What are the motivating factors for joining the nursing profession?
4 To what extent do nursing students and nurses draw upon rule-based, utility-based and virtue-based reasoning in responding to ethical dilemmas, and what does this tell us about the current ethical state of nursing?
5 What hinders or helps nurses in exhibiting virtuous practice?
6 What recommendations can be given to nursing educators about improving the teaching of professional ethics in the field?

As explained in the project's final report (Kristjánsson, Varghese *et al.*, 2017), the study was explicitly motivated by the assumption that nurses require a range of moral virtues as well as the capacity to exercise good judgement. In turn, a further assumption motivating the study was that preparing nurses ethically and educationally for the challenges of the profession is conducive to both their own flourishing and the well-being of their patients. With these assumptions in mind, the study aimed at ascertaining a better understanding of the ethical terrain of the nursing profession and the ways in which new entrants to the nursing profession are prepared for the ethical challenges they are likely to encounter. The project's research design incorporated self-reporting measures of personal and professional character, as well as ethical dilemmas and interviews with nurses at different stages of their careers and with nursing educators. The project comprised a mixed-methods, cross-sectional design. This design enabled the project team to examine: (1) what nursing students, experienced nurses and nurse educators *said* about character and nursing; (2) how considerations to do with character influenced nursing students' and experienced nurses' thinking about *moral dilemmas* in nursing; and (3) the *contextual* factors that may shape and influence the character of nurses.

Adopting a mixed-methods design, the study involved surveys and interviews. To test the feasibility of the survey, a hardcopy survey was piloted with 25 nursing students at the University of Birmingham. The main aim of the pilot study was to test the survey and to identify and resolve any potential problems or issues, especially with the presented ethical dilemmas. Following the delivery of the pilot survey, an open session was held with the research team, where students were invited to discuss and resolve any issues that they had encountered when taking the survey. Apart from minor amendments to occasional terminology, the survey was considered ready to be administered to the larger group.

In the main study, the survey was administered to first-year and final-year nursing students at seven UK universities and to nursing practitioners with more than five years of experience. Experienced nurses were identified and recruited through the alumni offices of participating universities, as well as via NHS Trusts. The survey was completed online and in hard copy (where online was inconvenient). In total, 696 participants completed the survey. As presented in Table 0.1, the distribution of completed surveys was evenly split among the three cohorts, permitting generalisations to be made and conclusions to be drawn within and across each cohort.

Table 0.1 Survey and Interview Participants

Career Stage of Participants	Number of Completed Surveys	Number of Interviews Conducted
First-year students	230	24
Final-year students	249	24
Experienced nurses	217	26
Educators	N/A	10
Total	696	84

The questionnaire consisted of the following five sections.

Section A – Ethical dilemmas: In this section, respondents were presented with six ethical dilemmas, similar to those used in the previous research by the Jubilee Centre (see Arthur, Kristjánsson, Thomas *et al.*, 2015; Arthur, Kristjánsson, Cooke *et al.*, 2015). Ethical dilemmas were used in this and other studies on professions conducted by the Jubilee Centre as they (1) offer a potentially credible way to gain an insight into moral functioning and development and (2) can be designed to activate more than simply moral reasoning skills, namely, moral motivations as clues to potential moral action (Kristjánsson, 2015b: chap. 3). Nevertheless, responses to dilemmas serve as an indication, rather than guarantee, of action or understanding of moral sensitivity in a real, particular situation. They do not, in and by themselves, *measure* virtue, nor do any such definitive measures exist elsewhere, but when combined with data from interviews and self-reports, they may contribute to an overall understanding of virtue in professional practice. The dilemmas each explored the role of character and virtues in decision-making processes in clinical settings and were designed by a panel of experts drawn from the four main specialities of nursing education, that is, adult, children's, learning disability and mental health.

Section B – Your character strengths: This section consisted of a list of 24 VIA-IS character strengths derived from the Values in Action inventory (Peterson and Seligman, 2004; Peterson and Park, 2009). Respondents were given the opportunity to consider their own character strengths and to choose and rank six strengths, which best described the sort of person they are.

Section C – About you: Respondents were asked a set of demographic questions as well as to disclose the current stage of their education (students) or area of practice and experience in years (practitioners).

Section D – Your work environment: The questions in this section elicited respondents' views regarding their work or study environment (only final-year students and practitioners, as the first-year students were yet to begin their initial practice placement). This section adapted questions from a Europe-wide workplace survey (Eurofound, 2012) with additional questions on ethical issues in the workplace.

Section E – 'Ideal' nurse: Respondents were asked about their views on the character strengths of an 'ideal' nurse. Here, they were asked to identify and rank six character strengths from the 24 VIA-IS character strengths to 'best describe a good nurse', followed by an open question asking to describe their reasons for choosing the nursing profession.

As stated earlier, the survey data were complemented by 74 semi-structured interviews,[3] conducted with a selection of respondents (at least 10%

from each group; see Table 0.1) who had indicated a willingness to be interviewed when completing the survey. In addition, interviews were conducted with ten nursing educators. These latter interviews explored how nursing educators conceived their role in educating future nurses; how they assessed students for entry onto undergraduate courses; their views of a good professional in their field; how this view might have changed in the course of their career; whether the character strengths required for good nursing practice might change and why they might do so; what informed their teaching in relation to the virtues; and how much the NMC Code of Conduct influenced their teaching. Most of the interviews were conducted face to face and lasted for approximately 30–45 minutes. Where in person interviews were not possible, telephone interviews were undertaken. All interviews were recorded, with the audio recordings transcribed, and returned to participants for member checking to allow for amendments and to ensure that transcription provided a fair reflection of what the participant wanted to convey.

Data from undergraduate students were collected at University of Birmingham, Birmingham City University, Buckinghamshire New University, University of Dundee, Manchester Metropolitan University, University of Northampton and University of Greenwich. Students were contacted by email and provided with a link to the survey by the contact lecturer at each university and through each university's online learning platform. The research team visited each site and introduced the project through lectures where students were given the opportunity to participate. A proportion of the data was collected via traditional pen-and-paper methods where email or online response was not deemed practical. The experienced professionals were contacted initially through alumni offices at the University of Birmingham, University of Dundee and Buckinghamshire New University. Due to a low rate of initial responses, Chief Nurses/Heads of Nursing at hospitals and NHS Trusts across the United Kingdom were approached in order to request participation from nursing staff. Once the agreement was in place, all nurses in each Trust were sent an invitation via NHS email requesting voluntary participation. Flyers were put up in departments to advertise the project, and paper copies were handed out to be distributed to nurses who preferred to complete the survey on paper.

Turning to the analysis of the data, data collected on paper surveys were entered into a database and then transferred to SPSS, version 23, to be checked, cleaned and readied for analyses. Data collected via the online survey were exported to SPSS, version 23, and followed the same process. Analyses included descriptive analysis, cross-tabulation and correlation. Analyses were also developed to deal specifically with the results of sections on respondents' views on character and ethical dilemmas.

The analysis of interview data was thematic, using a constant comparison method (Glaser and Strauss, 1967). A modified framework approach was adopted for this (Ritchie and Spencer, 1994). The research team independently analysed the data from the interviews and developed the themes and categories. Categories were refined, and coding was reviewed throughout the process.

Limitations and ethical considerations

As stated in the final report of the *Virtuous Practice in Nursing* project (Kristjánsson, Varghese *et al.*, 2017), certain limitations relating to the study should be pointed out. First, the study was cross-sectional. Whilst a longitudinal design would have been ideal to chart the *development* of character through nursing education and practice, the time that it would have taken to track nursing students from university entry to experienced practice excluded the possibility of such a design. Furthermore, due to possible variations in the membership of the three cohorts studied, questions may be raised about exact comparability between the groups. A further limitation is response bias. More generally, surveys of character (like personality testing more generally) suffer from self-report and social desirability biases. Involvement in the study was voluntary, and full participation by all who were invited to respond could not be ensured. That meant that only those participants who were disposed favourably enough to the topic (whatever their views on it) responded. Consequently, the survey and interviews represented the views of a self-selected group of people and not a perfectly unbiased sample.

The study received ethical approval from the University of Birmingham Ethics Committee. Some of the participating universities also gained approval via internal committees. Ethical approval from the NHS was not required for participating experienced nurses, as there was no discussion of patients or patient data. The research participants were fully informed of the scope and methods of the research through an information leaflet before participating. Once participants had read the information sheet and given full consent to participate, they had the right to withdraw within up to six months after the data collection phase had been concluded. Participants' confidentiality was protected by anonymising survey responses and interview transcripts.

The structure of this book

Following the introduction, this book comprises four main chapters and a conclusion which contains a summary of the main findings, recommendations and areas for further research. Chapter 1 presents a brief review of current literature in the wider field of professional ethics. Arguing that the ethical dimension is central to what is meant by a profession, Chapter 1 introduces the recent turn to virtues and character within the literature on the professions, in particular the focus on *phronesis* (practical wisdom). In this context, the Jubilee Centre's *Building Blocks of Professional Practice* are also introduced. In Chapter 2, attention turns to the ethical nature of the nursing profession. Here, we contend that, as with professions more generally, the ethical forms a fundamental component of what it is that constitutes the 'good' nurse, with a specific focus on virtue ethics and the concept of *phronesis* or professional wisdom. Surveying current literature in the field, the chapter also highlights some impacts on the ethical nursing of increased marketisation and instrumentalism within healthcare systems.

In Chapters 3 and 4, data from the *Virtuous Practice in Nursing* project introduced earlier are presented and analysed. In Chapter 3, data are examined to consider how the nursing students and experienced nurses in the study conceived character in relation to the role of the nurse and to nursing as a profession more widely. The data presented provides an initial snapshot of the motivations of the respondents to enter the nursing profession and the sort of nurse (in terms of character, rather than specialism) they wished to be when embarking on their career. In addition, the chapter also presents data regarding how respondents across the three career stages conceived their own personal character strengths as nurses and those character strengths they identified with the 'ideal' or 'good' nurse. The chapter also examines data setting out how the respondents in the study understood the varied contextual factors that enabled and constrained their ability to practise professional virtue in their workplace settings.

In Chapter 4, we analyse responses to the series of ethical dilemmas given to the nursing students and experienced nurses in the study. On the basis of associations made by the expert panel, we focus on three dilemmas to analyse the type of reasoning – virtue-based, ruled-based, or consequence-based – selected most commonly by respondents. The chapter also considers the data across the six dilemmas employed in the study to analyse the reasons prioritised across the cohorts. Finally, the chapter explores key themes raised in the interviews with experienced nurses and medical educators, particularly with regard to how ethics is included and encountered their respective experiences of nursing education. This book ends with *Conclusions, Recommendations and Further Research*.

Our intention in the pages that follow is to bring together data, analysis, findings and conclusions from the *Virtuous Practice in Nursing* project in order to consolidate and share with new audiences what the project revealed about the ethical dimensions of nursing practice and nursing education and to open up areas for further investigation that might shape the research trajectory over the coming years.

Notes

1 The professional regulator for nurses and midwives in the UK and for nursing associates in England.
2 www.jubileecentre.ac.uk/1595/projects/virtues-in-the-professions
3 A copy of interview schedule can be found at www.jubileecentre.ac.uk/nursing

1 The professions and character

Introduction

Whether inspired by a desire to justify an occupation's status as a profession (e.g., teaching and social work) or by the need to re-assert precisely what lies at the heart of a long-standing profession in the wake of public concerns about standards (e.g., medicine and law), the related questions of what constitutes a profession and what constitutes professional practice have received a great deal of attention over recent years. A core concern within this literature on the professions has been to highlight and seek to understand the ethical basis of professions, whether generally or specifically. Professions are deemed inherently ethical occupations because, and more so than other occupations, they place high moral demands on the conduct of workers. Indeed, these ethical and moral demands – which include care, integrity, fairness and diligence – are often viewed as *the defining* feature of many professions, including nursing, medicine, law and teaching, reminding us that professions are ultimately concerned with *human* actions and interactions. As Oakley and Cocking (2001) remind us, the focus of professional work is typically the provision of goods – such as health, education and justice – that are fundamental to flourishing individuals and societies. In specific relation to healthcare, a number of authors cite the importance of virtues such as trust, compassion and kindness as being core to the profession (see, e.g., Tuckett, 2000; Armstrong, 2006, 2007; Brody and Doukas, 2014; Rhodes, 2020). Yet, and as various professional 'scandals' over the last 20 years have evidenced, every profession and professional faces ethical challenges and dilemmas as part of their work. Indeed, the very ethical nature of the professions entails that public mistrust and criticism results when conduct falls below the standards expected (Blond *et al.*, 2015).

In order to examine the ethical nature of professions and the ethical dilemmas experienced by professionals, since its inception, the Jubilee Centre has

DOI: 10.4324/9781003146308-2

undertaken a number of empirical studies examining character, virtues and the professions. Some of these studies have concentrated on the professions generally (Arthur *et al.*, 2019), while others have focused on specific professions: law (Arthur *et al.*, 2014), medical practice (Arthur, Kristjánsson, Thomas *et al.*, 2015), education (Arthur, Kristjánsson, Cooke *et al.*, 2015), business (Kristjánsson, Arthur *et al.*, 2017) and the British Army (Arthur *et al.*, 2018). More recently, through the project *Practical Wisdom and Professional Practice: Integration and Intervention*, the Centre has built on this research to examine particular commonalities and differences across professions and professionals (Arthur and Earl, 2020).

The purpose of this chapter is to provide an initial survey of the existing literature on the professions. The first section considers briefly what constitutes a profession in general terms, before turning to the more specific ethical dimensions of professional activity. It does so in light of the now widespread trend towards managerialism, accountability and efficiency, which has been witnessed across professions in a number of countries over the last 30 years. In the second section, attention moves to consider the value of a virtue-based account of professional ethics. In this section, we draw on the Jubilee Centre's neo-Aristotelian approach to virtues and character in order to argue that professional ethics not only involves but also transcends reliance on rules and duties, thereby requiring professionals to act with professional wisdom and judgement.

What constitutes a profession?

While definitions of what constitutes a profession abound, certain features seem to be generally, if not universally, accepted (see, e.g., Carr, 1999). These are that:

- a profession is a paid occupation;
- a profession requires formal qualifications, a high level of education and a prolonged period of training/induction;
- a professional possesses high level theoretical and practical expertise in a given discipline;
- a profession provides a public service;
- a profession is, and professionals are, held in high esteem within society;
- a professional acts with integrity, care, honesty and trust, exhibiting a level of professional autonomy and judgement;
- professional ethics is guided by a code of conduct specific to that profession.

The Australian Council of Professions,[1] which captures each of these features, define a 'Profession' as follows:

> a disciplined group of individuals who adhere to ethical standards and who hold themselves out as, and are accepted by the public as possessing special knowledge and skills in a widely recognised body of learning derived from research, education and training at a high level, and who are prepared to apply this knowledge and exercise these skills in the interest of others. It is inherent in the definition of a Profession that a code of ethics governs the activities of each Profession. Such codes require behaviour and practice beyond the personal moral obligations of an individual. They define and demand high standards of behaviour in respect to the services provided to the public and in dealing with professional colleagues. Further, these codes are enforced by the Profession and are acknowledged and accepted by the community.

In the United Kingdom, various professions make clear the centrality of the 'ethical' to the nature of the profession. For example, in its Code of Ethics,[2] the British Association of Social Workers asserts that:

> Ethical awareness is fundamental to the professional practice of social workers. Their ability and commitment to act ethically is an essential aspect of the quality of the service offered to those who engage with social workers. Respect for human rights and a commitment to promoting social justice are at the core of social work practice throughout the world.

The Law Society of England and Wales[3] makes clear that:

> The commitment to behaving ethically is at the heart of what it means to be a solicitor.
>   Ethics is based on the principles of:
>
> • serving the interests of consumers of legal services
> • acting in the interests of justice acting with integrity and honesty according to widely recognised moral principles
>
> Ethics will help you respond in the right way to any moral dilemmas you might face at work.

Many more codes of conduct from other professions that similarly locate ethical conduct as fundamental to the profession could be cited. However, despite these reasonably well-established and understood definitions, how best the ethical should be formulated conceptually and can be implemented practically, remains both disputed and challenging.

Clearly, ideas about what constitutes the 'good' professional transcend simply technical abilities and encompass notions of judgement, wisdom and care. However, further questions remain about the extent to which particular cultures, discourses and practices can put pressure on how professionals, particularly those working in the public sector, can act with (or indeed without) ethics and integrity (see, e.g., Furlong *et al.*, 2017). Indeed, various studies evidence the impact (whether positive or negative) of workplace conditions on professionals' ability to exhibit ethical conduct (see, e.g., Oakley and Cocking, 2001; RPS, 2011; Worth and Van Den Brande, 2019).

Discussions about the meaning and nature of ethical professional conduct and the effect of cultures, discourses and workplace practices typically concentrate around two particular considerations. The first is the impact, widely cited and critiqued in the current literature on ethics and the professions, of the increased forms of managerialism and instrumentalism that have roundly been identified as detracting from the ethical and societal role of professionals. According to critics, the turn to managerialism across and within the professions has led not to a renewed form of professionalism but to a processes of de- and re-professionalisation through which the goals of general accountability (to service-users and to government) and efficiency have actively worked against professional autonomy and judgement (Carr, 2011; Holbeche and Springett, 2004; George, 2017). The second consideration is the extent to which professions, such as health, teaching and social work, have come under increased public scrutiny and accountability in the wake of various 'scandals' (Seijts *et al.*, 2017). Over the last 25 years in England, for example, high profile cases including the murder of Stephen Lawrence and resulting Stephen Lawrence Inquiry (known commonly as the Macpherson Report), the murder of Victoria Climbié, the death of Peter Connelly (also known as Baby P), the Mid Staffordshire hospital crisis and the Rotherham Child Sexual Exploitation scandal have all raised serious questions about what were significant failures in professionals' ethical judgement and conduct.

In the context of managerialism, accountability, efficiency, public scrutiny and increased workplace pressures, professions and professionals need to (re)envisage the ethical nature of their work. This (re)envisaging by necessity includes paying attention to what a profession aspires to be, what constitutes professional practice – whether generally or specifically for that profession – and how external factors shape the standing and work of professions today. In the next section, we start to examine these questions through a focus on a virtue-based approach to professional ethics. In doing so, we introduce key work in the field, particularly that makes reference to the concept of professional *phronesis*.

A virtue-based approach to professional ethics

The last few decades have witnessed a groundswell of interest in virtue-based approaches to professional ethics. Though not the only variant of a virtue-ethical approach, the majority of this interest has drawn on Aristotelian roots, and this concerted interest in Aristotelian/neo-Aristotelian virtue has been applied across a range of professional contexts, including accountancy (e.g., West, 2017), medicine (e.g., Pellegrino and Thomasma, 1993), nursing (e.g., Armstrong, 2006, 2007), social work (e.g., Adams, 2009), and youth work (e.g., Bessant, 2009). In particular, two Aristotelian ideas have provoked significant interest among those concerned with professional ethics. The first is the idea that virtues represent 'contextually appropriate traits . . . such as honesty, compassion and perseverance' that contra rules 'become habitually ingrained through deliberate and repetitive practice, predisposing practitioners to behave based on ethically sound habits' (Arthur *et al.*, 2019b: 2). The second idea – the main focus of this section – is the concept of *phronesis*, or practical wisdom (Pellegrino and Thomasma, 1993; Gillies, 2005; Kinsella and Pitman, 2012; McKie *et al.*, 2012). It is important to note, however, that while often cited, *phronesis* is not understood *uniformly* throughout the literature on professions (for a useful overview of *phronesis* in nursing, see Jenkins *et al.*, 2019). Indeed, examining work on *phronesis* in professional medical ethics, Kristjánsson (2015a: 299) highlights the 'considerable lack of clarity in the current discursive field on *phronesis*'.

In line with its neo-Aristotelian philosophy, the Jubilee Centre advocates the following model of the *Building Blocks of Professional Practice* (see Figure 1.1).

In Figure 1.1, *phronesis* – or practical wisdom – is defined as 'the overarching meta-virtue, developed through experience and critical reflection, which enables a professional to perceive, know, desire and act with good sense. This includes discerning, deliberative action in situations where virtues collide'. In other words, professionals need a certain form of practical wisdom, or *phronesis*, which can be defined in the following way:

> To practice with *phronesis* is to act with care, diligence and open-mindedness. To practice without *phronesis* would mean acting carelessly, indecisively, and with a degree of negligence to the surrounding circumstances or possible consequences.
>
> (Arthur *et al.*, 2019b: 5)

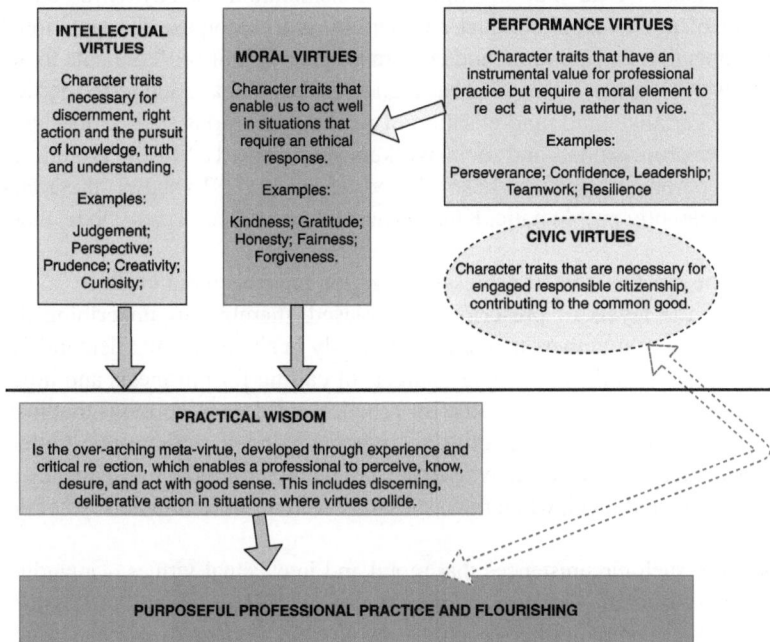

Figure 1.1 The Building Blocks of Professional Practice

The Jubilee Centre's *A Framework for Character Education in Schools* (2017), adapted to a professional domain. The model depicts the four domains of virtue and their conceptual relationship with practical wisdom and the purposeful professional practice.

For some authors, it is possible and useful to identify a form of professional *phronesis* – or what Sellman (2009: 1) terms the 'professionally wise practitioner'. Sellman (2012: 116) defines the professionally wise practitioner as one who:

> continually strives to be the best practitioner she or he can be given the constraints under which practice occurs. For practitioners, this endeavor includes but is not restricted to understanding the limits of their own personal professional competencies together with a willingness to identify and work toward rectifying relevant competency deficits. These are demanding requirements that imply a deep understanding of the turbulent and dynamic nature of practice, a recognition of the value of some form of critical self-reflection, and a resolve not to allow complacency to jeopardise future practice.

Sellman makes clear that an important consideration for any virtue-based account of professional conduct and activity is to recognise the situational constraints that can act upon and constrain the ability of professionals to act ethically. As Pitman (2012: 131) has argued, and as we have suggested earlier, the managerialism and marketisation of public professions such as teachers, healthcare professionals and social workers have created a 'hostile ground for growing phronesis' (see also Dixon-Woods *et al.*, 2011). To neglect these factors is inherently problematic. Kinsella and Pitman (2012: 8) remind us that:

> as the mechanisms of professionalization have been put in place, so too have the levels of prescription increased, thereby circumscribing the capacity of members to act autonomously in situations that demand the exercise of judgement. The 'danger' of calling for phronesis and holding practitioners accountable for practical wisdom in contexts that may not support it, and that actively mitigate against it, is that practitioners may face a double bind, where they are blamed for a failure of agency at the personal level, when the issues may well be structural and systemic.

It is under such circumstances that moral and intellectual virtues – including the meta-virtue of *phronesis* – play a crucial role, enabling professionals to discern and deliberate about the correct course of actions given the *salient features at play* (Russell, 2009). Indeed, initial findings from a meta-analysis of professional virtues undertaken by the Jubilee Centre (Arthur *et al.*, 2019a: 5) indicate that the '*phronetic* professional is one that is posited to endorse both moral and intellectual virtues in conjunction with one another'. These initial findings suggest 'the importance of developing a *phronetic* character profile for the enhancement of perceived professional purpose. That is, one that encompasses a value for both moral and intellectual virtue simultaneously as opposed to in isolation of one another'. Importantly, moral virtues may be crucial for developing a sense of purpose that extends beyond the self to the community in which one works', but 'it is only when a moral compass is synergised with a valuation of the intellectual virtues, that professionals are likely to experience the greatest possible sense of professional purpose' (Arthur *et al.*, 2019a: 16). In other words, moral and intellectual values work together to guide the right action and a deeper sense of professional worth.

Codes of conduct and the limitations of rule

A core feature of professional occupations, then, is the ability to handle the ethical dilemmas and challenges faced within the workplace. Professional work is such that, given the complexity of their work and challenges involved in delineating an ethically appropriate course of action, the professional cannot simply follow given guidelines or codes – particularly when ethical requirements conflict (e.g., when loyalty conflicts with honesty). So too, and given the complex nature and scope of professional activity, the professional must draw on a range of salient information – theories, practices, prevalent codes, relationships involved and potential outcomes – to discern the right course of action for the right reasons (see, e.g., Fish and de Cossart, 2013). In certain circumstances, the complexity and challenges of their occupation may place professionals in situations where their actions may be both morally right and yet run counter to the requirements set out by government and related agencies (Moore, 2015). As Carr (1999: 35) contends, 'responsible professional decisions must depend ultimately on the quality of *personal* deliberation and reflection'.

This is not to suggest, however, that the sort of practical wisdom needed for professional *phronesis* can be completely separated from the principles and rules that often characterise professional codes of conduct (Pellegrino and Thomasma, 1993). Having a clearly stated set of principles and rules brings a number of benefits in terms of educating new entrants to the profession, guiding professional conduct and providing those external to the profession (patients, clients, parents, pupils, etc.) with some understanding of what can be expected of the profession concerned. However, rules and codes of conduct can only help the professional so far and are insufficient for true ethical practice if they are not accompanied, interpreted and balanced by intellectual and moral character. In simple terms, where codes of conduct are too rigid, cultures of conformity can undermine professional autonomy and judgement; where codes of conduct are overly ambiguous, they offer professionals little by way of structure and guidance to act as a basis for their deliberations and choices.

Rules, then, may well form part of characterising ethical professional practice, but in and of themselves, they are an insufficient basis for true ethical practice if they are not accompanied, interpreted and balanced by intellectual and moral character. American psychologist Barry Schwartz has spoken about the ways in which the dominance of external controls, such as rules and incentives, can actively *undermine* wisdom and judgement. According to Schwartz (2009):

> rules and incentives may make things better in the short run, but they create a downward spiral that makes them worse in the long run. Moral skill is chipped away by an over-reliance on rules that deprives us of the opportunity to improvise and learn from our improvisations. And moral will is undermined by an incessant appeal to incentives that destroy our desire to do the right thing. And without intending it, by appealing to rules and incentives, we are engaging in a war on wisdom.

Importantly for the focus of this book, Schwartz (2011) has also argued that the dominance of rules and incentives does not only limit professional wisdom but also serve to undermine professional motivation. He argues that:

> the problem with relying on rules and incentives is that they demoralize professional activity, and they demoralize professional activity in two senses. First, they demoralize the people who are engaged in the activity. Judge Forer quits, and Ms. Dewey in completely disheartened. And second, they demoralize the activity itself. The very practice is demoralized, and the practitioners are demoralized. It creates people – when you manipulate incentives to get people to do the right thing – it creates people who are addicted to incentives. That is to say, it creates people who only do things for incentives.

The *phronetic* professional, then, is not guided solely by duty to codes external to their own intellect and morals or by externally driven incentives, but rather conceives and applies their professional responsibilities by using their professional wisdom. This includes the understanding codes of conduct, but not conceiving these as the sole arbiter when dilemmas arise. As the author C. S. Lewis (1985: 100; cited in Bohlin, 2005: 20) eloquently wrote in his *Letters to Children*:

> A prefect man would never act from a sense of duty; he'd always want the right thing more than the wrong one. Duty is only a substitute for love (of God and other people), like a crutch, which is the substitute for a leg. Most of us need the crutch at times; but of course its idiotic to use the crutch when our legs (our own loves, tastes, habits etc) can do the journey on their own.

Lewis' words remind us that sound professional conduct has have an internal motivation and meaning – and that is, it must come from the heart. It is for precisely this reason that many, if not all, professions are understood as vocations rather than simply occupations.

Focusing on the sorts of capacities frequently associated with professional *phronesis*, which include sensitivity, discernment, deliberation and reflection, signifies that the codification of professional conduct into a set of rules cannot be disentangled from the critical judgement of the professional. Indeed, the critical judgement of the professional is crucial if those rules are to be applied in practice and in a way that juggles the demands of the specific situation at hand (including where stated rules may be in conflict). Whether one subscribes to an Aristotelian notion of *phronesis* that separates ethical from technical practice or from a MacIntyrean approach that understands technical practice to have an ethical dimension, it remains that the ethical is core to professional practice (Cooke and Carr, 2014; Kristjáns-son, 2015b; Kotzee *et al.*, 2016).

Conclusion

In this chapter, we have surveyed existing literature on the ethical dimensions of professions. As we have intimated in this chapter, it is not a question of *whether* professions such as medicine, law, nursing, social work and teaching involve an ethical dimension but rather how this dimension is and should be conceived and enacted by these professions. While general approaches to professional ethics act as a significant starting point in responding to these latter questions, the nature, demands and realities of professional ethics are necessarily moderated by the particular profession at hand. In other words, while we might approach the general ethical dimensions of professions from a given framework (in the case of the Jubilee Centre, a broadly neo-Aristotelian one), it is also necessary to appreciate that the precise ethical demands that act upon doctors, nurses, lawyers, teachers and so on are likely to be framed and expressed in ways particular to those individuals' professions. With this in mind, the next chapter focuses more specifically on ethics and nursing.

Notes

1 www.professions.com.au/about-us/what-is-a-professional
2 www.basw.co.uk/about-basw/code-ethics
3 www.lawsociety.org.uk/support-services/ethics/

2   Virtues and the ethical nurse

Introduction

Nursing is an essentially ethical profession. When we think of what it means to be a nurse, we think readily of nurses who are kind, caring and compassionate. Yet, despite the enduring ethical nature of nursing as a profession, the contours of nursing ethics – particularly how ethical codes and conduct are, and should be, applied in practice – remain dynamic and subject to discussion. Indeed, recent years have witnessed ongoing debate about the ethics of nursing, whether focused on the most appropriate theoretical frameworks for conceiving nursing ethics, on the relative roles of codes and/or professional judgement by nurses in practice or, indeed, on concerns about the actual conduct of nurses in particular contexts. The idea, which we pursue in this book, that nursing requires particular moral dispositions is fairly commonplace within the existing literature, with much pointing to the idea that patients need to have confidence in a 'good' nurse who possesses personal qualities such as compassion, patience, trustworthiness, honesty and kindness. In turn, the expression of these qualities can be viewed as crucial for enacting good quality decision-making and care (Poorchangizi et al., 2017; Armstrong et al., 2000). As Florence Nightingale[1] suggested:

> Nursing is an art: and if it is to be made an art, it requires an exclusive devotion as hard a preparation as any painter's or sculptor's work; for what is the having to do with dead canvas or dead marble, compared with having to do with the living body, the temple of God's spirit? It is one of the Fine Arts: I had almost said the finest of Fine Arts.

Recent research suggests, however, that while nurses are cognisant of the ethical dimensions of their profession, and often seek to promote ethical practice in their work, questions remain about the confidence and ability of nurses to enact professionalism fully. These concerns, as we make clear in

DOI: 10.4324/9781003146308-3

this chapter, are connected to a range of factors, including whether nurses have sufficient education and professional development about ethical nursing, whether nurses have sufficient autonomy in their work and whether structural and contextual barriers in healthcare systems and settings actually preclude nursing with character. In this chapter, we offer a narrative review (we do not claim this to be a comprehensive review given the space possible) of existing literature on nursing ethics, focusing specifically on virtues and character. Following others, we understand nursing as an essentially ethical profession and nursing as a moral enterprise (Carr, 1999). As such, our interest here is on the ethical dimensions of nursing and the role of the nurse. This chapter comprises two main sections. In the first section, we offer some overview analysis of nursing as a profession, before examining two particular and relevant factors that have for some time been impacting on how nursing professionalism is understood and practiced – the marketisation of healthcare and levels of trust in nursing as a profession. In the second section, our focus moves to the character of nurses. Here, we consider more specifically the appeal of virtue-based approaches to conceiving and framing nursing ethics, including the key role identified for the meta-virtue of *phronesis*.

The professional ethics of nurses in context

Nursing is a profession rooted in professional ethics and ethical standards, and nursing practice is, or at least should be, guided by such ethical standards. How well nurses are able to practice ethically impacts on the quality of healthcare received by patients, and such practice needs to be guided by a level of professional judgement through which nurses are able to prioritise amongst competing pressures. Of fundamental importance, here, is the idea that nurses advocate for their patients, placing the needs and interests of patients at the heart of their care (Tuckett, 2000; Tollefsen *et al.*, 2021). Viewed as a moral way of being, nursing historically has had its focus on the wellness of others and with nurses being connected with their patients through caring and trustful relationships (Gilligan, 1982). The moral formation necessary to this conception of nursing as a profession comprised part of the education of nurses from the very beginning of nursing schools in England from the 1860s, and this trend continues today. As stated in the introduction to this book, the Nursing and Midwifery Council's[2] (NMC, 2020: 6) code of professional standards of practice and behaviour emphasises the need to 'prioritise people', to 'treat people as individuals and uphold their dignity' and to 'treat people with kindness, respect and compassion'. Indeed, in the most recent iteration of the Code, the NMC makes clear their commitment that the Code serves to reinforce the professionalism of nurses. To quote directly from the Code, various aspects of professional conduct and practice are detailed, including that to 'uphold the reputation of the profession' nurses must:

- keep to and uphold the standards and values set out in the Code;
- act with honesty and integrity at all times, treating people fairly and without discrimination, bullying or harassment;
- be aware at all times of how your behaviour can affect and influence the behaviour of other people;
- keep to the laws of the country in which you are practising;
- treat people in a way that does not take advantage of their vulnerability or cause them upset or distress;
- stay objective and have clear professional boundaries at all times with people in your care (including those who have been in your care in the past), their families and carers;
- make sure you do not express your personal beliefs (including political, religious or moral beliefs) to people in an inappropriate way;
- act as a role model of professional behaviour for students and newly qualified nurses, midwives and nursing associates to aspire to.[3]

Within the field of nursing ethics, debate continues to abound about whether the ethical practice of nurses is best understood through rule-based, consequence-based or virtue-based approaches and, more aptly, about the relative merits and relations between the three. It is important to note from the outset, of course, that while the qualities required of nurses might be easily stated, the actual work of nurses occurs within complex and dynamic healthcare settings. Moreover, this work and these settings operate within particular regulatory, political, economic and social contexts, each of which shape not only the intentions and meaning of the qualities (e.g., what it means to be compassionate, what is understood by professional autonomy or judgement) but also the ability of nurses to live up to the high ethical standards expected (or at least desired). As such, any meaningful account of the ethics of nursing as a profession must engage with both the structures and the conditions within which nurses practice and how ethics are – and could be – understood and enacted in actual clinical settings.

So far as this first task is concerned, two factors are of particular importance, whether for our own purposes in this book or for the field more widely. The first factor is that the healthcare needs of the United Kingdom's population and the environments in which care is provided and delivered are changing rapidly. Though the actual changes involved differ between the four nations of the United Kingdom, the National Health Service in England has been subject to ongoing major structural and financial change over the last 40 years. Such change, whether for good or ill, has come in the context of persistent uncertainty about the ability of the National Health Service to meet the demands placed upon it, whether now or in the future. More specifically, the marketisation of healthcare and the increased levels of managerialism within healthcare settings have altered the way in which nurses and other healthcare professionals work – including how they relate to their patients. As Armstrong (2006: 112) has argued in relation to a helping relationship between nurses and patients characterised by kindness and patience:

> this kind of helping relationship is only achievable if nurses make themselves available to patients, spend sufficient time with patients, and listen attentively to what patients have to say. Unfortunately, literature suggests that nurses are spending most of their time on administrative tasks and only a small proportion of their time is spent in direct contact with patients.

Similarly to other professions, the marketisation and managerialism encountered by the nursing profession have led to higher levels of scrutiny and accountability of both individual nurses and nursing as a profession, with some even claiming that nursing itself has become a 'marketable commodity' (Foth and Holmes, 2016; Kim *et al.*, 2015; George, 2017; Mercile, 2018; Lipscomb, 2019). With specific regard to nursing in England, concerns continue about whether the rhetoric of compassionate care both for and by nurses will be, or indeed can be, realised in practice given the 'political ideology that drives healthcare in the UK' (George, 2017; see also Flynn and Mercer, 2013). As Foth and Holmes (2016: 7) point out, the changes to healthcare organisation and provision have also impacted on nursing education, with a shift identified towards competency-based education. For these authors, the impact has been to move nursing education to 'be tailored according to the demands of employers, administrators, or the market by redefining or cutting those competencies no longer considered necessary'.

A second factor, one not unrelated to the first, of particular importance regarding the wider context within which nurses work is the standing of the profession with the wider public. While studies suggest that public trust in nurses remains high, several high-profile incidents have brought the quality of nursing care into sharp focus. In England, and with regard to the former, the 2019 Ipsos Mori (2019) *Trust in Professions Survey* found that nurses remain the most trusted profession, with 95% of respondents stating that they trusted nurses to tell the truth. Conversely, several high-profile scandals and subsequent reports have placed a focus on the provision of healthcare, including by nurses. The Report of the Mid Staffordshire NHS

Foundation Trust Public Inquiry Executive summary (Francis Report) published in February 2013 firmly suggested a need for increased quality in the ethical conduct of nurses and nursing as a profession, arguing a need for an increased culture of compassion and caring in the recruitment, training and education of nurses. The report states, for example, that patients were treated with 'callous indifference' (Great Britain. Parliament. House of Commons, 2013: 13). Francis is also reported to have stated that 'there was a lack of care, compassion, humanity and leadership' at the Trust (*The Independent*, 7 February 2013). In addition, the report called for a consistent standard for nurse education – a task since taken up by the Nursing and Midwifery Council (2019).

As was suggested in the book on the medical profession in this series, a notable educational challenge of the current context is for the nursing profession and for nurses to operate within a wider culture of higher expectations, wider responsibilities and the pressures of marketisation. It is precisely these cultures that, at the same time, place significant pressure on nurses to enact their professional character – to be compassionate in their care of patients, for example – while also necessitating greater levels of professional character (e.g., working in multi-disciplinary terms, handling uncertainty, balancing competing pressures). The point we are making here is that nurses have to aspire to excellence within workplace contexts that while not wholly constraining, do place pressures on the capacity to provide compassionate care and which serve to limit the flourishing of nurses, other healthcare professionals, patients and other stakeholders.

Nurses of character

The ideas of moral character and virtue have received some significant attention within the literature on nursing ethics over the last 30 years (Tuckett, 2000; Armstrong, 2006, 2007; Banks and Gallagher, 2009; Gallagher, 2020; for some more cautious or critical accounts of the move to virtue in nursing ethics, see Holland, 2010; Newham, 2015). As has already been suggested previously in this book, so far as nursing is concerned moral character and virtue are intertwined with the somewhat broader idea of the 'ethic of care'. The 'ethic of care' is not defined by a set of rules or principles, but rather is a way of practicing that requires specific moral qualities that enable nurses to enact the caring relationship with patients, and to do so through informed judgement (Tronto, 1994; Vanlaere and Gastmans, 2007). Corley (2002) notes that because nurses act as moral agents within a connected healthcare system, the patient, nurse and organisation all benefit from nurses' moral acts. Such acts, which may require a degree of moral courage, include those in which nurses act as advocates for their patients, interpreting the needs of the patient to other members of the multidisciplinary team and to patients' families. Writing some 15 years ago, and reiterating a point raised in the previous section, Nathaniel (2006) raised concerns about the complexity – including the emotional sensitivity – of healthcare environments. In such circumstances, the ability to promote an ethic of care is affected by factors beyond the nurse's control. More positively, a number of scholars have pointed to the mutual reinforcement gained through nursing directed towards human flourishing (see, e.g., Sellman, 2011; Ahlstedt *et al.*, 2020). The contention is that through a commitment to understanding the vulnerability of the patient and the desire to promote the patient's flourishing, the nurse's own character not only comes to the fore but can also be further developed.

While to some extent a response to principle- or rule-based approaches to nursing ethics, the focus on virtue-based approaches to nursing ethics within the academic literature resonates with some core directions of travel within nursing itself. NHS England's (2012: 13) Vision and Strategy for Nursing, Midwifery and Care staff titled *Compassion in Practice* further embedded the principle of the following 6Cs as forming the 'enduring values and beliefs that underpin care wherever it takes place':

Care

Care is our core business and that of our organisations, and the care we deliver helps the individual person and improves the health of the whole community. Caring defines us and our work. People receiving care expect it to be right for them, consistently, throughout every stage of their life.

Compassion

Compassion is how care is given through relationships based on empathy, respect and dignity – it can also be described as intelligent kindness, and is central to how people perceive their care.

Competence

Competence means all those in caring roles must have the ability to understand an individual's health and social needs and the expertise, clinical and technical knowledge to deliver effective care and treatments based on research and evidence.

Communication

Communication is central to successful caring relationships and to effective team working. Listening is as important as what we say and do and essential for 'no decision about me without me'. Communication is the key to a good workplace with benefits for those in our care and staff alike.

Courage

Courage enables us to do the right thing for the people we care for, to speak up when we have concerns and to have the personal strength and vision to innovate and to embrace new ways of working.

Commitment

A commitment to our patients and populations is a cornerstone of what we do. We need to build on our commitment to improve the care and experience of our patients, to take action to make this vision and strategy a reality for all and meet the health, care and support challenges ahead.

Nurses, of course, grapple with different kinds of practice dilemmas on a day-to-day basis – and a core interest within virtue-based accounts of nursing ethics is how nurses handle the various ethical decisions faced in their clinical practice. While not wishing to discount the value of codes of conduct (such as the NMC's Code), virtue-based accounts point to the importance of nurses' character, including their judgement or professional wisdom (to which we will return later), in mediating situations in which different courses of action are available and in discerning the right course of action. In other words, while any meaningful account of nursing ethics must pay due recognition to the codification of standards of conduct, such codification cannot provide all of the necessary ethical resources required by nurses to act with an ethic of care. A further point to note here is that one possible implication of a principle-based, rather than character-based, approach to the ethics of professional practice is that codes of conduct can also encourage an attitude of *compliance*. As Campbell and Chin (2011: 1–2) suggest:

> familiarity or even an ability to recite the entire ethical code and ethical guidelines without missing a punctuation mark does not guarantee ethical conduct and professionalism. Internalisation of the profession's moral edict has to take place before it can manifest as attitudes and behaviour.

Similarly, and with specific regard to nursing, Armstrong (2006) points out that an obligation does not exist nor does it do anything in isolation, a person needs to conceive, interpret and apply the obligation to others in morally complex situations.

If we move the focus briefly to the education and professional development of nurses, the associated argument becomes clear. Namely, that the formation of ethically good nurses cannot be focused narrowly on knowledge and adherence to a given code of conduct or principles, nor even with wise reasoning about such principles. Instead, the ethical development of professions must also include the nurturing of character, including the opportunity to engage in critical and collaborative dialogue and reflection on what it means to care, to be compassionate and so on, as well as on real-life complexities experienced in clinical practice. Vanlaere and Gastmans (2007: 764) have written about the importance of 'critical companionship' for the professional education of nurses, arguing that:

> The overall purpose of critical companionship is to enable nurses to practice in ways that are person centred and evidence based. It combines the expressive and intuitive processes of relationships and creativity with rational processes of analysis, critique and evaluation of practice and its knowledge. Role modelling, the exploration, articulation and critical reflection on skills and knowledge considered as taken for granted, enable nurses to become reflective practitioners.

It should be remembered here, too, that viewing nursing ethics from the perspective of the moral character of nurses resonates with understandings of what motivates people to become nurses (Wu *et al.*, 2015). Yet, ongoing concerns have been expressed in different contexts about whether the education of nurses actually attends to the encouragement of internalised character traits in an intentional and comprehensive way (see, e.g., Grady *et al.*, 2008; Sellman, 2011; Kinsella and Pitman, 2012; Krautscheid and Brown, 2014; Hoskins *et al.*, 2018).

While standards can – and do – incorporate core qualities needed by nurses, they remain a step detached from the complexities of clinical practice and cannot provide the nurse with a guide to moral action in each and every situation experienced – such a resource needs also to come from within. This stated, the importance within virtue-based accounts of *phronesis* – that is, of *professional wisdom* or *good judgement* – as an educable virtue comes to the fore. On a broadly neo-Aristotelian view of character, *phronesis* is the integrative, meta-virtue that enables the professional to perceive, know, desire and act with good sense (there is no space in this chapter to provide a full account of the conceptual discussions of *phronesis* in the literature on nursing ethics; for a detailed consideration see, Jenkins *et al.*, 2019). Generally, and for our purposes here, professional wisdom enables nurses to discern the morally salient features of the situation and factor these into their clinical decisions alongside the range of other variables and conflicts, avoiding excess and deficiency. As Sellman (2011: 174) contends, the nurse who practices with professional *phronesis* is one who when faced with a set of guidelines can:

> choose from a range of possible courses of action. Thus she or he will need to remain open to a number of possibilities including: the possibility that the protocol may be in need of revision; the possibility that she or he may be wrong to follow the protocol in general; and the possibility that she or he may be wrong to follow the protocol in any particular instance.

It is through professional wisdom that nurses are best able to respond to the various contextual features of a given situation, while seeking to preserve the ethic of caring for their patient(s). As with virtue-ethics more widely, this specific focus on *phronesis* in nursing is now reasonably long standing (Kelly, 1993; Bishop and Scudder, 1996; Gastmans *et al.*, 1998; Van Hooft, 1999; Armstrong, 2006; Haggerty and Grace, 2008; Sellman, 2011; McKie *et al.*, 2012; Jenkins *et al.*, 2019; Ko *et al.*, 2020).

For advocates of virtue-based approaches to professional ethics, this contextual adaptability is of fundamental importance. One particular relevance of attention on professional wisdom – and the formative processes required to support it – is the connections with the ongoing interest in nursing ethics about how nurses can find it difficult to respond in an appropriate way to situations of moral conflict and, as a consequence, how they can experience intense moral distress (Edmonson, 2010; Fourie, 2015; Ko *et al.*, 2020). Research has suggested that the moral distress experienced by nurses can often result from a conflict between the professional and personal desire to care and the constraints of the work environment. Jameton (1984), for example, framed the concept of moral distress as arising when one knows the morally right thing to do, but cannot enact this due to organisational constraints, conflicting values and the beliefs of other healthcare providers. Repenshek (2009) reported that continuing conflict can eventually lead to chronic stress for patient care providers (see also Butterworth *et al.*). These latter reflections remind us that paying attention to nurses' character and decision-making in specific contexts speaks in important ways to the realities of clinical practice, including within multidisciplinary settings. Moreover, some researchers have contended that ethical conflicts in clinical settings are increasing due to a range of factors (see, e.g., Pavlish *et al.*,

2014; Hoskins *et al.*, 2018). With these reflections in mind, there is at least a possibility that the development of *phronesis* by nurses – particularly if that development occurs within and through an environment of dialogue, reflection and collaboration – might serve to reduce levels of moral distress. In turn, a fundamental question remains as to how professional wisdom might best be developed through nursing education, with some suggesting that rather than being developed through direct teaching, professional wisdom needs to be cultivated through careful, attentive and reflective processes (Haggerty and Grace, 2008; McKie *et al.*, 2012).

Conclusion

In this chapter, we have sought to provide an overview, though not an exhaustive account, of the extant literature on nursing ethics, with a particular focus on virtue-ethics. Our suggestion in this chapter, following others, is not that codes of professional standards for nurses are not important, nor that they say nothing at all about the qualities required by nurses – including the need for developing and employing professional judgement. Here, the NMC Code provides a case in point. We have cited core aspects of the Code so far, but here we point to the fact that in being built around the four principles of prioritising people, practising effectively, preserving safety and promoting professionalism and trust, the Code requires nurses to use their professional judgement (and indeed a whole range of qualities of character) to enact its provisions. Given this, and the associated and more general point that codification cannot ever provide all of the moral resources necessary for professional ethics in practice, attention has rightly been paid to the importance of cultivating the character of nurses. Crucial to this is the recognition that nursing is an act and practice of care, constituted by deep moral relationships between nurses and their patients that, when enacted well, involves virtues such as compassion, honesty, trust and kindness. Understanding nursing ethics in this way brings into focus the character of nurses, and the sorts of nurse they wish to be – a question that cannot be wholly divorced from either nurses' own personal character or the complex, and often challenging, settings in which nurses engage in their clinical practice. As such, the meta-virtue of phronesis – or professional wisdom – plays a crucial role in enabling the good nurse to discern, deliberate about and pursue the right course of action in morally and medically complex situations. We move now to present and analyse the empirical data developed in the *Virtuous Practice in Nursing* study in order to explore how nurses at various stages of their careers conceive their own character and that of the 'ideal' nurse, as well as the sorts of reasoning these nurses drew upon when presented with a series of ethical dilemmas.

Notes

1   https://resources.nurse.com/nightingales-quotes-2020
2   The professional regulator for nurses and midwives in the UK and for nursing associates in England.
3   www.nmc.org.uk/standards/code/read-the-code-online/

3 Nurses and nursing

Motivations, personal character strengths and ideal character strengths

Introduction

Recalling that a general aim of the *Virtuous Practice in Nursing* project was to build up a picture of the role of character strengths and virtues in the professional lives of nurses by exploring them from a number of different angles, in this chapter we present, analyse and discuss empirical data drawn from the Jubilee Centre project – *Virtuous Practice in Nursing* (Kristjánsson, Varghese *et al.*, 2017) – which examined how the nursing students and experienced nurses in the study understood character in relation to the nursing role and to nursing as a profession more widely. This chapter consists of three main sections. In the first section, data presented provide an initial snapshot of the motivations of the respondents to enter the nursing profession and the sort of nurse (in terms of character, rather than specialism) they wished to be when embarking on their career. The second section presents data regarding how respondents across the three career stages conceived their own personal character strengths as nurses and those character strengths they identified with the 'ideal' nurse. In the third section, we analyse character and virtue in context. Here, we present data setting out how respondents understood the contextual factors that enabled and/or constrained their ability to practise professional virtue in their workplace settings. These responses are classified into four main headings: autonomy, involvement, support and challenge. By exploring these themes, we consider the key features of the workplace that influence virtuous practice, at least as far as the respondents in this study were concerned.

Personal motivations and virtues

We start the presentation and discussion of the findings of the *Virtuous Practice in Nursing* study by considering the data regarding respondents' motivations for entering the nursing profession. In the survey, respondents

DOI: 10.4324/9781003146308-4

were presented with an open-ended question about these motivations, while the semi-structured interviews each commenced with the question: 'Why did you choose nursing as a career?'

Analysis of the survey and interview data evidenced, unsurprisingly, that multiple factors influenced beginning and experienced nurses' decision to enter the profession. This said, one theme – providing caring for others – stood out as what the original project team referred to as a 'master-theme'. In the responses, the motivation to care for others manifested in various ways. Within the open-ended question in the survey, many respondents spoke of *nursing as a vocation* that either they had chosen or, for some, that had chosen them. Closely connected with the idea that nursing was a vocation was that the caring and altruism that stand as the (real or perceived) defining features of nursing corresponded to the sorts of character traits respondents entering the profession held important and/or wanted to develop. The **desire to 'care for' and 'help'** others were commonly mentioned within the surveys and interviews. One survey respondent stated that they '*felt it [nursing] was a job well suited to my character and a job that would give me real enjoyment and satisfaction*', while one final-year student explained:

> I want to be the person that sits on the end of someone's bed and comforts them when they're going through a tough time, and be there for support. It's just one of those things that I just knew I wanted to do and it's all I wanted to do.
>
> (Final-Year Student)

Although the main reference to caring was directed towards other people, in some responses, the object to which care was directed either was or included the current state of the National Health Service. Surveys responses to this end included the following:

> I chose the nursing profession as there is a large margin for improvement in the NHS and I hope to help end the stigma surrounding minority patients. I also believe it will be hugely rewarding and allow me to exercise my best qualities plus better myself.

> I decided to become a nurse as I want to be part of the NHS's future. I want to help promote good health . . . and also help an individual maintain their health whatever their health status may be.

Often connected with the notions of caring for and helping others was a personal connection or experience that had served to spark or cement the motivation to enter the nursing profession. A number of respondents to the survey referenced the care they had observed and experienced, either to themselves or close family members. Indeed, the role modelling of care by others was also a theme conveyed in the interviews, as the following extracts illustrate:

> My sister has a disability, she has cerebral palsy, and she was in hospital when we were younger, and I was with her in hospital. When I went to visit, and go in, I'd see the nurses and they were always just amazing, and they always helped. So, it stemmed from there, I think.
>
> (First-Year Undergraduate Student)

> I think it all came from an episode I had in hospital when I was about 14 years old. That opened my eyes to nursing; I'd never contemplated it before that. So, it was a personal experience, I feel.
>
> (Experienced Nurse)

> It was something I always wanted to do personally. My mum's a nurse but it wasn't primarily because of that, it was because when we were growing up my younger brother was quite ill – he had cancer – and he was treated at a local hospital. So it was something that I always wanted to do after that.
>
> (Experienced Nurse)

Interestingly, however, there were a few instances in which *negative* experiences of nursing were cited as a motivation for becoming a nurse (referred to by the original project team as 'reverse emulation'). As one experienced nurse recounted:

> I had a personal experience where I had to go to hospital – not quite an emergency, but an acute episode. And at the time there was a nurse there, and I didn't feel she was particularly caring or supportive when I was there. And I always thought, 'Do you know what? I could do better than her'.

Closely connected to the role-modelling of care observed and experienced in clinical settings was that provided by other family members who were nurses, and who had inspired respondents to become nurses themselves. Numerous respondents referenced how they had grown up in a family where at least one close relative was a nurse and that this has played a pivotal part in motivating their decision to be a nurse. One experienced nurse, for example, spoke of how her family contained 'nine nurses' and that, as a result, 'family conversations were always about nursing'. Similarly, a final-year undergraduate student reported:

> I had aunties who did nursing, I had cousins who did nursing, every-body in my family did nursing, so it was always going to be something I did.

Alongside these caring-focused motivations stood several other more instrumental or perhaps immediate impetuses that had led some respond-ents to enter the nursing profession. In the interviews, one experienced nurse explained 'I went into nursing because I wanted to leave home and I wanted a career which gives me accommodation and a job', while another suggested:

> I didn't set out to be a nurse, and I didn't . . . I wasn't a child that always had a career path, but when I left school I was in . . . I think I did a secretarial course for about a year and I wasn't satisfied, and I knew I wanted something else. And my friend was applying for nursing, so I applied at the same time.

While for another experienced nurse:

> I wanted to be efficient and I guess I wasn't really ever signed up to be one of those weeping, hand-holding nurses really, I was always much less about the kind of, you know, the Florence Nightingale and much more about the efficient and professional nurse really. I was never, I think because I had a very realistic view of nursing, because my entire family came from nurses, I didn't have a romanticised idea of nursing at all. I knew it was a hard slog, with lots of ups and downs and so I was very realistic about it, I think, far more realistic than other people in my position were.

Of course, the fact that the initial motivation to become a nurse was not motivated strongly by a desire to care for and help others does not neces-sarily entail that such a desire did not materialise through the processes of becoming and being a nurse.

Moving now to the personal virtues reported in the survey, in the project, and mirroring the approach taken in other projects focusing on professions conducted by the Jubilee Centre, respondents were provided with a list of 24 character strengths from which to choose to describe their own per-sonal character and that of the ideal doctor (from Peterson and Seligman's

Character Strengths and Virtues Classification, 2004). Respondents were asked to rank the six character strengths they thought best reflected their personal character as nurses. Among all of the respondents, five character strengths were most commonly identified:

- kindness
- honesty
- teamwork
- fairness
- humour

Further to these five strengths, which were common across the three career stages included in the study, there were slight differences in the sixth personal character strength cited most commonly between student nurses and experienced nurses. While love was one of the six most common personal character strengths identified by students, experienced nurses reported leadership as their sixth personal character strength. Indeed, while love was the sixth highest preferenced/ranked character strength for both first-year and final year undergraduate students, it was only the 17th highest preferenced/ranked character strength for experienced nurses. While experienced nurses preferenced/ranked leadership as the 6th highest character strength, this was preferenced as the 12th highest by first-year undergraduate students and as the 8th highest by final-year undergraduate students. Across the three cohorts appreciation of beauty, zest and prudence were the least reported character strengths. Table 3.1 illustrates the total percentages of the three most reported and three least reported character strengths by each cohort.

Table 3.1 Personal Character Strengths Across Cohorts (%)

Personal Character Strengths	First Year (%)	Final Year (%)	Experienced Nurses (%)
Kindness	17.1	17.7	14.4
Honesty	15.0	16.1	17.1
Fairness	8.5	8.5	12.4
Appreciation of beauty	0.7	0.9	0.4
Zest	0.2	0.6	0.4
Prudence	0.7	0.1	0.3

    Highest preference/ranking

    Lowest preference/ranking

Table 3.2 Personal Character Strengths Ranking by Cohort

Personal Character Strengths	Ranking		
	First Year	*Final Year*	*Experienced*
Kindness	1	1	2
Honesty	2	2	1
Fairness	3	4	3
Teamwork	4	3	4
Humour	5	5	6
Leadership	12	8	5
Love of learning	9	10	7
Perseverance	7	11	9
Curiosity	8	9	12
Love	6	6	17
Social intelligence	11	13	13
Forgiveness	13	7	20
Judgement	14	19	8
Perspective	16	16	10
Hope	18	12	14
Creativity	15	15	16
Bravery	10	17	21
Gratitude	17	14	19
Self-regulation	21	19	11
Spirituality	19	21	15
Modesty	20	18	18
Appreciation of beauty	22	22	23
Zest	24	23	22
Prudence	22	24	24

Table 3.2 presents the ranking of the personal character strengths. Table 3.3 presents the total scoring of the top six personal character strengths reported across all cohorts.

The data collected through the interviews with respondents from all three cohorts provide further depth into these personal character strengths. Of course, the interviews enabled respondents to cite a wider range of character strengths – indeed virtues – than those found in the VIA classification. The most commonly cited within the interviews were compassion, care, humility, patience, perseverance, integrity and honesty. This simple identification aside, the interview data provide insights into how these concepts were understood and applied by respondents, including how different virtues can

Table 3.3 Top Six Personal Character Strengths Across All Cohorts

	Personal Character Strength
1	Kindness
2	Honesty
3	Fairness
4	Teamwork
5	Humour
6	Leadership

work alongside or, indeed, how they might conflict. An illustrative example here is honesty. Within the interviews, respondents spoke of the need for honesty with themselves, with their colleagues and with their patients. In addition, some respondents spoke of honesty in relation to what might also be termed integrity and as involving standing up for what they believed to be right. Interview data, too, highlighted the processes and conditions perceived to be important in cultivating and sustaining the personal character strengths central to nursing. Experienced nurses interviewed, for example, suggested that personal character strengths need to be nurtured and mastered in and through practice. In this regard teamwork, support from within the working environment and positive role models were all cited by experienced nurses as playing an important role in the professional development of good nurses. We say more about the role of teamwork and support in the third section and more about the educational importance of positive role models in the next chapter.

Virtues of the 'ideal' nurse

In the survey, the same 24 character strengths were presented to the respondents who were asked to rank the six they thought best captured the character strengths of an 'ideal' nurse. Analysis of these responses again evidenced some important commonalities, with all cohorts reporting kindness and honesty as either the first or second most important character strength of the ideal nurse. More specifically, first-year undergraduate students ranked kindness as the most important, whereas final-year students and experienced nurses ranked honesty as the top character strength. Across all three cohorts, the following four character strengths completed the top six highest preferenced/ranked:

- teamwork
- fairness

Table 3.4 'Ideal' Character Strengths Across Cohorts (%)

'Ideal' Character Strengths	First Year (%)	Final Year (%)	Experienced %
Kindness	18.3	15.9	17.8
Honesty	15.7	17.9	17.9
Teamwork	11.8	12.6	12.7
Zest	0.2	0.4	0.6
Appreciation of beauty	0.2	0.5	0.3
Spirituality	0.1	0.4	0.3

         Highest preference/ranking
         Lowest preference/ranking

- leadership
- judgement

There was, then, firm agreement across all cohorts on the top six ideal strengths, with only a slight variation in the ranking order. The three lowest preferenced/ranked character strengths respondents identified in the ideal nurse were zest, appreciation of beauty, and spirituality. Table 3.4 illustrates the total percentage of preferences for the three highest and three lowest preferences/rankings. Table 3.5 shows the ranking of the 'ideal' character strengths by each cohort. Table 3.6 displays the total scoring of the top six 'ideal' character strengths reported across all cohorts. Spirituality, appreciation of beauty and zest were the three least important strengths ranked between the three cohorts.

Within the interviews, it was the student nurses who spoke at most length about the character strengths of the ideal nurse. Once again, interview settings enabled respondents to make reference to a wider set of strengths than those found within the VIA and to do so with more nuance. Some respondents highlighted in the interviews that the ranking task in the survey was difficult given both that all strengths were important and that different situations call for different strengths. For example, a final year undergraduate student reflected:

> Definitely being kind and caring, I think, would come at the top of the list. Then honesty definitely has to be one. And humour, I think. More so because I think humour's important everywhere because I think without it we'd always just be quite upset about things. It can really be quite therapeutic when applied appropriately. Leadership, I think,

Table 3.5 'Ideal' Character Strengths Ranking by Cohort

'Ideal' Character Strengths	Ranking		
	First Year	*Final Year*	*Experienced*
Honesty	2	1	1
Kindness	1	2	2
Teamwork	3	3	3
Fairness	4	5	4
Leadership	7	4	5
Judgement	6	7	6
Bravery	5	6	11
Humour	10	10	8
Love of learning	13	8	7
Perseverance	9	15	9
Hope	14	9	12
Love	8	12	16
Perspective	12	11	15
Self-regulation	15	13	10
Social intelligence	11	14	14
Curiosity	16	16	12
Creativity	18	18	17
Forgiveness	20	17	20
Gratitude	17	19	21
Prudence	19	24	18
Zest	23	22	19
Modesty	21	20	24
Appreciation of beauty	22	21	23
Spirituality	24	23	22

being a nurse is definitely a privileged position and using that position with good leadership I think can allow not only yourself and your colleagues and your patients, but everyone to flourish and do better. I think judgement is definitely quite key. It's something you have to use in your assessments of someone. You have to use it in day-to-day life, your judgement of individuals, and your judgement of conditions.

Interesting too are the similarities and differences between these top six strengths of the ideal nurse and those presented earlier regarding the

Table 3.6 Top Six 'Ideal' Character Strengths Across All Cohorts

Ideal Character Strength
1 Honesty
2 Kindness
3 Teamwork
4 Fairness
5 Leadership
6 Judgement

personal strengths as nurses reported by respondents. Five virtues – kindness, honesty, fairness, leadership and teamwork – appear in the top six of both. In the character strengths respondents associate with the ideal nurse, however, humour is replaced by judgement. Table 3.7 presents a comparison in rankings between the personal and 'ideal' character strengths split across each cohort.

As we have mentioned earlier, other studies conducted by the Jubilee Centre on different professions have captured the comparison between personal and 'ideal' character strengths. Table 3.8 presents a comparison between five professions in this regard: business and finance, nursing, medicine, law and teaching.

As Table 3.8 demonstrates, there is a close similarity – one not always found in the other professions – between the three highest preferred/ranked character strengths of the 'ideal' nurse and their own reported character strengths. Once again here, and as testified to within the interviews, we can see the close connection between personal characteristics and motivations and those perceived (by the respondents and more widely) as being fundamental to good nurses and nursing as a profession. One further point of analysis is that, and in somewhat of a contrast to teachers in the Centre's *The Good Teacher* study, non-moral virtues (or better, strengths) received less attention. While in the survey, as it drew on the VIA list of character strengths, this might be explained by the measure itself (the VIA includes perseverance but not, for example, resilience or determination), these non-moral virtues did not surface to the extent one might have expected. Generally, where resilience was mentioned by the experienced nurses, it was in general terms either in an expression that the respondent saw themselves as being resilient or that the demands of nursing required a certain degree of resilience. Within these responses there was a sense that the non-moral strengths were important in enabling ethical conduct (in the sense that a nurse needs to be resilient if they are to be able to practice with compassion and kindness), but the nature and universality

Table 3.7 Comparison between Personal and 'Ideal' Character Strength Rankings for Each Cohort

	First-Year Ranking		Final-Year Ranking		Experienced Ranking	
	Personal	'Ideal'	Personal	'Ideal'	Personal	'Ideal'
Kindness	1	1	1	2	2	2
Honesty	2	2	2	1	1	1
Appreciation of beauty	22	22	22	21	23	23
Teamwork	4	3	3	3	4	3
Love of learning	9	13	10	8	7	7
Social intelligence	11	11	13	14	13	14
Fairness	3	4	4	5	3	4
Perspective	16	12	16	11	10	15
Zest	24	23	23	22	22	19
Perseverance	7	9	11	15	9	9
Creativity	15	18	15	18	16	17
Gratitude	17	17	14	19	19	21
Love	6	8	6	12	17	16
Hope	18	14	12	9	14	12
Leadership	12	7	8	4	5	5
Prudence	22	19	24	24	24	18
Modesty	20	21	18	20	18	24
Humour	5	10	5	10	6	8
Self-regulation	21	15	19	13	11	10
Spirituality	19	24	21	23	15	22
Curiosity	8	16	9	16	12	12
Forgiveness	13	20	7	17	20	20
Judgement	14	6	19	7	8	6
Bravery	10	5	17	6	21	11

Highest correspondence between rankings

Lowest correspondence between rankings

of this connection between the respondents were not something that came through with full clarity. We cannot rule out that this was a result of the questions asked, but it does raise an area where further research would be insightful.

Table 3.8 Top Three Personal and 'Ideal' Character Strengths, Combining All Cohorts for Each Profession

Character Strengths	Business and Finance	Nursing	Medicine	Law	Teaching
Top 3 'personal' character strengths	Honesty Fairness Teamwork	Kindness Honesty Fairness	Fairness Honesty Kindness	Fairness Honesty Humour	Fairness Honesty Humour
Top 3 'ideal' character strengths	Leadership Judgement Teamwork	Kindness Honesty Teamwork	Fairness Honesty Judgement	Judgement Honesty Perseverance	Fairness Humour Love of learning

Virtues of the nursing profession: the importance of context

As widely noted, and as we suggested in Chapters 1 and 2, professional virtues always sit within a given context. Whether it be the immediate context of the workplace setting, the wider contexts of policy, healthcare systems and public discourse, or the extended contexts of family, peers and the media, context implicates how professionals act and practice. It is crucial, therefore, that any consideration of the importance of personal and moral dimensions of nurses pay particular attention to context. In this section, we draw upon two sources of data to explore the perceptions and accounts of context offered by respondents in the *Virtuous Practice in Nursing* study to explore the impact of work environment factors on actual nursing practice; these include the physical environment, organisational structures and resources.

As the student respondents surveyed in the project were either at the beginning or end of their initial nursing education, they were not included in this part of the survey. In other words, to understand context, only experienced nurses completed the specific section of the survey (Section D) relevant for this purpose. In Section D, respondents were presented with a 15-item questionnaire that explored experienced nurses' views of their workplace. These 15 items were classified into four factors (these factors were previously identified in the *Virtuous Medical Practice* report by the Jubilee Centre for Character and Virtues (Arthur, Kristjánsson, Thomas *et al.*, 2015: 24–26)), namely, 'autonomy', 'involvement', 'support' and 'challenges'. In addition, interview data with experienced nurses provide further insights into how context impacts – for good and for ill – on the professional character of nurses.

Table 3.9 Experienced Nurses' Views of the Degree of Autonomy They Are Accorded

Autonomy					
$N = 211$	Never	Rarely	Sometimes	Mostly	Always
Mean = 4.1	1	2	3	4	5
%	0	1%	5%	56%	38%

I am able to act in the best interests of my patients.
I have the resources to do my work to a standard I believe is right.

Autonomy

Of the 15 questions in the survey, the following two questions – 'I am able to act in the best interests of my patients' and 'I have the resources to do my work to a standard I believe is right' – were found to factor together. Some 211 experienced nurses responded to these questions and of those, 94% (38% *always* and 56% *mostly*) said they were able to practise autonomy in their workplace (see Table 3.9). Only 6% of nurses felt they were either *only sometimes* (5%) or *rarely* (1%) able to act as autonomous agents in their workplaces.

In the interviews, many respondents spoke of areas of their professional practice in regard to which they experienced autonomous agency and self-determination, including when making a patient assessment independently; when they make a clinical decision and clinical judgment which is right for the patient; and when they educate a patient. A common theme within these responses was that nurses indicated that they have a sense of autonomy and authenticity when acting as advocates of patients under their care. Generally, the experienced nurses interviewed were supportive of the principle of professional autonomy, equating this autonomy with a positive perception of the status of nursing – including in relation to other healthcare professions (most notably doctors). One experienced nurse identified the professionalisation of nursing as a positive change:

> I think the profession has changed . . . It has changed positively; we are seen in a greater professional manner by our medical and AHP colleagues. In a lot of circumstances, I think we are seen as equals within the multidisciplinary team rather than before when a consultant would go through the ward round and just leave a list of jobs for the nurses to do.
>
> (Experienced Nurse)

Similarly, another nurse explained in relation to evidence-based practice that:

> So, I think from that point of view, things are much better, much stricter on making sure that we are giving the best care but also keeping us right as professionals as well, we're making sure we are practising with what's the best practice for this patient. So I think professionally we can absolutely hold our head up high.
>
> (Experienced Nurse)

The following nurse connected the autonomy they experienced and practiced to the supportive environment in which they worked, in turn suggesting that the context was one that had enabled them to realise the value of their knowledge and practice:

> I was given the autonomy to make assessments and kind of develop into what the modern nursing field would like to be and what it strives for its students just now. What I mean is in the olden days, nurses were very much . . . you know, you used to hear people talk about nursing being the handmaiden, the doctors make the decisions and then the nurses do what they're told, whereas now, nursing I believe to be more of a profession in its own right with quite a distinct skill set and I think that . . . well, initially, my first job, I was given the autonomy and the confidence to be quite assertive and confident in what I was doing and I realised that my skills and my assessments and my specialities were different to others and just as valuable.
>
> (Experienced Nurse)

Not surprisingly given the concerns regarding the present conditions in which healthcare professionals work outlined in Chapters 1 and 2, the interviews also presented a picture of some concerns and constraints so far as the professional autonomy of the experienced nurses was concerned. Capturing a not uncommon concern, one experienced nurse commented: 'I think certainly the pressure on the NHS, the time constraints, have certainly made nursing a lot harder over the years'. Another spoke of the loss of professional voice that nurses and nursing had experienced, believing this to have been inhibited:

> I feel again that there has been a loss of confidence. I feel like nurses' voices aren't being heard as much now, so I think it makes it harder for nurses to feel that they are being listened to.
>
> (Experienced Nurse)

We return to the constraints alluded to here in more detail later in the chapter.

Involvement

To analyse the factor 'emotional involvement in work', the following three items in the survey were added together after factor analysis: 'I am emotionally involved in my work'; 'I have the feeling of doing useful work'; and 'I am motivated to work to the best of my ability'. Ninety-five per cent of the experienced nurses reported that they are *always* or *mostly* emotionally involved in their work as shown in Table 3.10, a level similar to those conveyed by experienced doctors – 98.2% – in the *Virtuous Medical Practice* study (Arthur, Kristjánsson, Thomas et al., 2015). Conversely, and notably, only 5% of the experienced nurses reported that they either *sometimes* (4%) or *rarely* (1%) felt involved emotionally in their work.

During the interviews, experienced nurses commonly explained that their emotional involvement in their work was connected to core virtues – such as compassion – and their sense of purpose. This connection is illustrated in the following extract, in which an experienced nurse positioned compassion as giving their work meaning and direction within the context of a challenging work environment:

> I think despite all the difficulties we have, I don't lose compassion. I mean, it's a difficult job because we are so short staffed, but compassion would be the last thing that would go.
>
> (Experienced Nurse)

A further matter in relation to involvement, and one which intersects with other themes identified here, was that certain relationships helped to sustain the work and emotional commitment of nurses. The following nurse,

Table 3.10 Experienced Nurses' Emotional Involvement in Their Work

Emotional Involvement in Their Work					
N = 214	Never	Rarely	Sometimes	Mostly	Always
Mean = 4.24	1	2	3	4	5
%	0	1%	4%	37%	58%

I am emotionally involved in my work.
I have the feeling of doing useful work.
I am motivated to work to the best of my ability.

for example, spoke about the sustenance they received from their positive interactions with patients and relatives:

> I think the biggest thing that keeps me going now is the feedback patients give me on an average day.
>
> (Experienced Nurse)

Important, too, was the view that positive relationships with colleagues in the workplace also helped to nurture and maintain emotional involvement. This was often framed around the idea that colleagues provided a role model, as expressed by this experienced nurse:

> I think positive role models make a big difference, when you see a nurse that's doing things how you think things should be done, and you model yourself on them.
>
> (Experienced Nurse)

These extracts highlight the relational nature of nursing as well as the role that positive relations with other actors – including patients and colleagues – play in supporting nurses to be able to practice and express their professional character. We turn now to consider this support in more detail.

Support

The following five items were combined to examine and understand the support nurses get from the work environment and which can be understood as facilitating virtuous practice: 'My colleagues help and support me'; 'I am treated fairly'; 'I am able to apply my own ideas in my work'; 'I am able to influence decisions that are important for my work' and 'I feel 'at home' in my workplace'. Taken together, 92% of the experienced nurses reported that they were *always* (33%) or *mostly* (59%) supported in the work environment, with only 8% of the experienced nurses reporting that they only received support from the work environment either *sometimes* (7%) or *rarely* (1%; as demonstrated in Table 3.11).

These factor scores were even higher than those obtained from the equivalent cohort of experienced doctors in *Virtuous Medical Practice* study (Arthur, Kristjánsson, Thomas *et al.*, 2015), suggesting that, according to these respondents at least, nursing in UK workplaces occurs within a supportive and collegial environment. Note here, too, that teamwork was ranked highly by the respondents as both a personal and an 'ideal' character strength of nurses. This is a notable finding given the continued concerns about shortages in staff, funding and time faced by the nursing profession – each factors

Table 3.11 Experienced Nurses' Views of the Supportiveness of the Work Environment

Supportiveness of Work Environment

$N = 213$	Never	Rarely	Sometimes	Mostly	Always
Mean = 3.87	1	2	3	4	5
%	0	1%	7%	59%	33%

My colleagues help and support me.
I am treated fairly.
I am able to apply my own ideas in my work.
I am able to influence decisions that are important for my work.
I feel 'at home' in my workplace.

that impact negatively on the qualitative experience of nursing (Kalisch *et al.*, 2010). Indeed, when we consider this point in light of the interview data what comes through is a picture that the support nurses gain from various sources enable them to continue their professional practice when feeling overstretched, overworked and undervalued. When asked about what kept them motivated in their professional practice, one nurse pointed to the *'good support from other nurses in the ward'*. Similarly, a nurse spoke of her work as a team leader and explained how caring for staff was a core aspect of their role, and how this in turn was beneficial for patients:

> Within the team itself I've got a more managerial role, as well, so I care about staff that I work with, the team. And not only gain good relationships with the staff, but ultimately improve standards for the patient, but also be sort of accepted as a team, part of their team, as well.
>
> (Experienced Nurse)

It is necessary to note, here, that the team within which nurses work does not consist simply of other nurses, but involves a range of other healthcare professionals and other workers. The importance of collegial multidisciplinary teams was also commented on by some of the respondents:

> I think nurses are very much like – it's like a family group on a ward situation. I think you learn from each other and I think that breadth of experience, not just from nurses but you gain so much from the other people. We spend a lot of time on, we had physios, OT, the medics doing, you know, treating people as a person and seeing the whole thing. It was the whole infrastructure around it that I think really helped in nursing.
>
> (Experienced Nurse)

The opportunity, often facilitated by colleagues, to engage in professional development was also identified by some of the experienced nurses as an important source of support. As a case in point, one nurse reflected:

> When I got my first staff nurse job, I had a senior charge nurse who was excellent at developing her staff and she saw people that were interested and motivated and one of the big things that's helped me in my career is that I was given the autonomy to kind of lead my own development.
>
> (Experienced Nurse)

Challenges

It would be unrealistic, of course, to paint a picture of the environment in which nurses work that is wholly positive. As we have covered in earlier chapters, a large body of academic and public literature attests to the often very challenging conditions of contemporary healthcare systems, including the NHS. Aside from the positive aspects covered so far in this chapter, respondents also spoke of some not insignificant challenges that manifest and that constrain their professional work. These challenges varied and included recent reductions in staff, heavier workloads and an increase in administrative tasks, each of which was positioned as keeping nurses away from patients' bedsides and as prohibiting the caring and emotional aspects of their work (as suggested by Armstrong, 2006). With regard to the survey data, the following five items factored together under the category 'challenges': 'My work involves tasks that are in conflict with my personal values'; 'My work requires that I hide my feelings'; 'I experience stress'; 'At work it is difficult to do the right thing' and 'I do not have time to do my work to a standard I believe is right'.

Only 17% of the experienced nurses said that it is *rarely* (16%) or *never* (1%) a challenge to live out their own character, as shown in Table 3.12. Starkly, an overwhelming majority reported that living out of their own character in their workplace was a challenge (83%), ranging between *always* (2%), *mostly* (18%) and *sometimes* (63%).

The idea of a constraining workplace environment was also conveyed by the experienced nurses in the interviews, with a picture often painted of issues such as pressures on time and staffing acting against nurses' moral obligations to their patients – though to different extents as the following extracts suggest.

Table 3.12 Experienced Nurses' Perceptions of Challenges to Living Out Their
Character

Challenges to Living Out Their Character

$N = 214$	Never	Rarely	Sometimes	Mostly	Always
Mean = 2.67	1	2	3	4	5
%	1%	16%	63%	18%	2%

My work involves tasks that are in conflict with my personal values.
My work requires that I hide my feelings.
I experience stress.
At work it is difficult to do the right thing.
I do not have time to do my work to a standard I believe is right.

Not all of the respondents presented the impact of the challenges faced
as being substantial in nature. One nurse, for instance, spoke in terms of a
'little bit of conflict' reflecting:

> I think sometimes your values not quite get lost, but when you're in an
> environment you have to incorporate the values as well, if that makes
> sense? And sometimes there might be a little bit of conflict. For exam-
> ple, you would always want to give as much time as possible to your
> patients and you're under time constraints. I think sometimes there may
> be a little bit of compromise.
>
> (Experienced Nurse)

This noted, for many respondents, the impact of the challenges faced was significant and deep seated. The following nurse, for example, depicted a deep
level of effect when explaining the pressures of working in a busy clinical area:

> And the consultant comes round or something like that, that's when the
> caring, compassion goes out the window, no matter what you're thinking.
>
> (Experienced Nurse)

Many nurses recounted instances when they had come away from patients
feeling that they did not do as much for those patients as their hearts dic-
tated, meaning that the patients did not receive the care they deserved. The
following two nurses explained this in relation to staffing pressures and the
management of beds, respectively:

> So the retention of staff is a continual barrier to actually working in the
> way that you would want to work.
>
> (Experienced Nurse)

> Constant bed managing that interferes enormously with being able to
> be compassionate. Being expected to move patients out of their bed and
> into the chairs, so that they can get the next patient into that bed. Mov-
> ing people late in the evening to the discharge ward when you know
> that that's not going to work and they end up coming back to you two
> days later because they never did get home. And, you know, we are not
> treating the patients compassionately when we do that. Collectively
> we're not. I don't believe I am, because I still do it with the concern that
> I . . . but the institution is making us behave in that way.
>
> (Experienced Nurse)

Perhaps the most concerning report from one of the nurses interviewed
involved the identification of bullying as a serious work environment concern, particularly when change is sought:

> Because you come up against quite a lot of bullying really, when you
> do try to make changes. And you can sort of see why people's attitudes
> change, and they think, I am not going to bother doing it anymore now,
> because you get complaints made against you.
>
> (Experienced Nurse)

As the extracts presented here illustrate, we can see that for these respondents, the workplace environment is often one that both supports and con-
strains their ethical professional conduct. These findings are consistent
with others studies on the nursing profession reviewed in Chapters 1 and 2.
While supportive colleagues and the opportunity to engage in meaningful
professional development were reported as core factors in enabling nurses
to express their character in their work, pressures of time, workload and
the management of patients were all identified as inhibiting experienced
nurses' ability to practice with care and compassion. Moreover – and cru-
cially given the importance of professional judgement and wisdom for a
character-based understanding of nursing ethics – the context described by
experienced nurses impacted on their autonomy to use their judgement. Yet,
here, differing accounts were offered. Some of the experienced nurses, as
the following two extracts suggest, spoke of the need to exercise professional judgement, something that they had space to do:

> I think we do have to do it a lot . . . there are situations where you are
> having to make professional decisions and judgements. And yes, you
> do need to make wise judgement – and I think that comes with experi-
> ence as well. You can't learn that overnight.
>
> (Experienced Nurse)

I think probably . . . you're able to exercise professional judgment a lot more yourself, now. It was very much well, certainly when I did my training, it was a very hierarchical structure, it was quite old fashioned I suppose you would call it now, which probably stopped you . . . I have to exercise professional judgement all the time.

(Experienced Nurse)

In contrast, other experienced nurses reported that the scope for autonomy and professional judgement had become reduced over time:

Actually I think in reality, our hands are much more tied now. And I think I had much greater autonomy when I first trained than I do now.

(Experienced Nurse)

I feel again that there has been a loss of confidence. I feel like nurses' voices aren't being heard as much now, so I think it makes it harder for nurses to feel that they are being listened to . . . I feel like respect for the nursing profession, there is an element now where there is not the same respect. You always feel that you have got to fight your corner; whereas before, the doctor would just say, 'Okay, I'll leave that to you because that's your job now.' And you got on with doing your job for the best of your patients.

(Experienced Nurse)

Conclusion

In this chapter, we have presented and examined data about what motivated nurses at different stages of their career to join the profession, as well as how they understand their own character strengths as nurses as well as those they position as being constitutive of the 'ideal' nurse. While unsurprisingly motivations to become a nurse varied, there was a strong sense in which providing caring for others stood out as a leading motivation. Moreover, it was notable that a number of respondents made clear connections between their own desire to care for others and the identification of nursing as a vocation defined by caring and altruism for others. The data evidenced that nurses across the three career stages prioritised certain core character strengths as representing their own personal character – kindness; honesty; teamwork; fairness and humour – as well as those they associated with the 'ideal' nurse – teamwork, fairness, leadership and judgement. When we turn to the workplace conditions reported by nurses, we are, as other research also suggests, presented with a somewhat mixed picture. The experienced nurses reported their desire to practice care, compassion and other character strengths within their daily work and spoke positively about the ways in which collegiality – including within multidisciplinary teams – acts to sustain the ethical professional practice. On the other hand, the experienced nurses also spoke to various degrees about the pressures that impacted their ability to provide the level of care, and indeed to enact character, within their workplaces. This latter point, while not necessarily novel, is important to state and recognise. Not least it connects with a further consideration – how experienced nurses respond to these pressures in the medium to longer term. Not all of the experienced nurses commented on this element, but we close this chapter with three extracts that provide food for thought about how nurses *are* responding positively given the pressures under which they work but which at the same time give room for some concern:

> I don't think anything has prevented me. I think it's about finding a way around things. I think sometimes you come up against obstacles like budgetary obstacles and things like that, but actually it's about doing the best that you can do with the resources that you've got and sometimes things can be very frustrating and we see that a lot now. The knock-on impact of poor staffing levels and things like that, but actually it's about doing the very best care that you can do for the people within the resources that you've got.
>
> (Experienced Nurse)

> I worry that lots of good nurses are leaving the NHS because the stress of a permanent fulltime NHS post means that you're stuck with mountains of paperwork – budgets, computer work, that pulls you away from patient care. I think there is very good care, and very genuine care being given throughout the NHS, but people are struggling to be able to deliver that in the way that they want to.
>
> (Experienced Nurse)

> A thing I like in nurses is we know it's difficult, but we never give up, and we always push ourselves to do more. But unfortunately that has a downside too, because people kind of know that, so they push us to the edge.
>
> (Experienced Nurse)

4 Nurses, ethical dilemmas and the ethical education of nurses

Introduction

Drawing on the data collected by the *Virtuous Practice in Nursing* study, analysis is presented of responses to a series of ethical dilemmas given to the medical students and experienced doctors. Across a number of Jubilee Centre projects, moral dilemmas have been used as a data collection tool (Arthur *et al.*, 2014; Arthur, Kristjánsson, Thomas *et al.*, 2015; Arthur, Kristjánsson, Cooke *et al.*, 2015; Arthur *et al.*, 2018; Kristjánsson, Varghese *et al.*, 2017; Kristjánsson, Arthur *et al.*, 2017). In the *Virtuous Practice in Nursing* study, participants responded to a set of professional dilemmas (six situational judgement tests (Patterson and Ashworth, 2011; Lievens and Patterson, 2011) designed by a panel of 11 experts in nursing education who adapted well-known dilemmas from the literature and designed a wholly new set of answer responses specifically for the study). As explained in the introduction to this book, dilemmas were used as they (1) promise to offer a credible way to gain an insight into moral functioning and development and (2) can ideally be designed so as to activate more than simply moral reasoning skills (Kristjánsson, 2015b: chap. 3). It is important to note here that responses to dilemmas serve as an indication, rather than guarantee, of action or understanding of moral sensitivity in a real, particular situation. They should not be viewed as a sole *measure* of virtue, nor do any such definitive measures exist elsewhere (Wright *et al.*, 2021). It is the case that when combined with data from interviews and self-reports, dilemmas may contribute to an overall understanding of virtue in professional practice.

The rationale for employing the six dilemmas, then, was to ask respondents to explain their reasoning and the judgements arrived at with a particular focus on virtue-based reasoning. It was hoped that the situational judgement tests would provide insights into (1) which character strengths are important in dilemma situations in nursing; (2) how they are important and (3) how they interact with other factors, such as explicit rules for nursing and the

DOI: 10.4324/9781003146308-5

consequences of certain decisions.[1] The use of dilemmas as a research instrument reflects the fact that 'professionals may face workplace dilemmas where they are required to make decisions that conflict with the desires of external agents' (Arthur *et al.*, 2019b; see also Moore, 2015). Dilemmas of the sort designed by the expert panel are a common feature of nurses' professional lives, and they involve complex matters that range in seriousness and may include matters of life and death. As such, nurses are required to possess and practice (or at least as we have suggested earlier, should possess and practice) certain core intellectual virtues commensurate with professional wisdom, including judgement/prudence and perspective, in order to discern the morally good course of action in the given circumstances (Carr, 2018). A core contention of the studies on the professions conducted by the Jubilee Centre for Character and Virtues is that considering dilemmas can offer important insights into how professionals engage with a given problem.

This chapter has two main sections. In the first section, we detail and analyse the findings in relation to three of the six dilemmas the student and experienced nurses were asked to consider. Based on the associations made by an expert panel, each of these three dilemmas provides an insight into the choices and reasons made by respondents. The analysis points not only to similarities across the three career stages in terms of the chosen courses of action but also to the prioritisation of different types of reasons between the dilemmas. We also look at the data across the dilemmas to consider the weighting given by participants to duty-based and virtue-based reasons. In the third section, we seek to add further depth to the analysis by exploring some implications that are raised for the education of nurses in light of the data presented in this and the previous chapters as well as additional data that are drawn from the interviews with nursing educators and experienced nurses.

Moral dilemmas and character strengths

In this section, we present and analyse the data obtained in relation to three of the six scenarios that were designed by an expert panel as 'situational judgement tests' to understand the relative use of virtue-based reasoning in the process of dealing with the ethical dilemmas. As with other studies conducted by the Jubilee Centre in relation to professional ethics, the research was interested in whether the virtue-based reasoning was distinct from reasoning that drew on deontological (rules and codes) and/or on the (real or perceived) best consequences. It is important to clarify here that the interest in analysing the situational judgement tests was not so much on the course of action chosen but was instead on the justifications (reasons) chosen by respondents. For the *Virtuous Practice in Nursing* study, and as we explain in relation to each dilemma explained in the following, respondents were given reasons for each of the two choices provided for each dilemma. The three dilemmas were those chosen by the original project team as providing the best illustration of how reasons associated with virtues, rules and consequences influenced the responses provided by nursing students and experienced nurses. To provide a brief synopsis of this choice, in the first dilemma we present, deontological reasoning was prioritised by respondents over consequentialist and virtuous reasons. In the second, the majority of the respondents identified virtuous reasons as their motivation to choose their preferred option. In the third, a conflict was found between duty-based and virtue-based reasoning among the respondents.

Dilemma elderly patient

The first dilemma we analyse here (which was Dilemma 1 in the original project report) asked respondents how they would respond to the following scenario:

> You are a staff nurse who enjoyed working in the elderly ward. But recently you feel the job is not as rewarding as it was before because new changes prevent spending much time with the patients. You are frustrated with your new conditions and feel sorry for the patients as sometimes the changes have compromised fundamental care. In the worst case, an elderly patient died without anyone around him. The management is ignoring all requests for more staff but subtly pressurising staff to manage with fewer staff so that they can meet their financial targets.

Having considered the scenario, respondents were given two possible options from which to choose. Option 1 was that they would just live with the new policies and attempt to operate as effectively as they can within them. Option 2 was that they would speak to their matron and alert higher authorities if things did not improve. Based on their choice of either Option 1 or Option 2, respondents were then asked to choose and rank the three best reasons for their decision from a choice of 6.

For those respondents who selected that they would just live with the new policies and attempt to operate as effectively as they can within them (Option 1), the following six reasons were offered:

> Reason 1: Things are like this everywhere and you are hopeful and optimistic that it will improve.

Reason 2: You do not believe that you will have any luck influencing management, so it is better to keep quiet.

Reason 3: You have a duty to continue helping your patients.

Reason 4: You want to avoid trouble for yourself or others.

Reason 5: You are a determined person and want to continue to be there for your patients as much as you can despite the forces working against you.

Reason 6: You are expected to follow management rules.

For those respondents who selected that they would speak to their matron and alert higher authorities if things did not improve (Option 2), the following six reasons were offered:

Reason 1: Everyone will be better off in the long run if you speak up.

Reason 2: You have a duty of care to your patients.

Reason 3: This is the compassionate thing to do.

Reason 4: If you or someone close to you were in the patients' position you would want the staff to take action.

Reason 5: You are a courageous person, and if there is a shadow of doubt in your mind about the care given, you will escalate your concerns.

Reason 6: If any more of these incidents happen, you will feel guilty.

Most respondents (92%) indicated that they would speak to the matron and alert higher authorities if things do not improve, with only 8% opting to just live with the new policies and attempt to operate as effectively as possible within them. Chart 4.1 shows the results for all participants. As the aim of the dilemmas as a research instrument was to show whether the reasoning informing each option relied on virtue-based, deontological or consequentialist considerations, and since only 8% of respondents chose Option 1, we chose here to examine the reasons selected by those respondents (i.e., the 92%) selecting Option 2. Here, the reasons selected prioritised those associated by the expert panel with duty-based reasoning over and above those the panel associated with virtue-based or consequentialist reasons.

Chart 4.1 displays the reasons selected by respondents at each career stage in terms of whether they selected virtue-based, consequence-based or duty-based reasons. As the chart makes clear, there was a notable degree of similarity across the career stages in terms of the type of reason selected. Forty-six per cent of first-year undergraduate students, 48% of final-year undergraduate students and 50% of experienced nurses prioritised duty-based reasons as their justification for selecting Option 2. A total of 2.28% of first-year undergraduate students, 30% of final-year undergraduate students and 29% of experienced nurses prioritised virtue-based reasons (which the expert panel associated with courage and compassion). As the original project team concluded, these results suggest

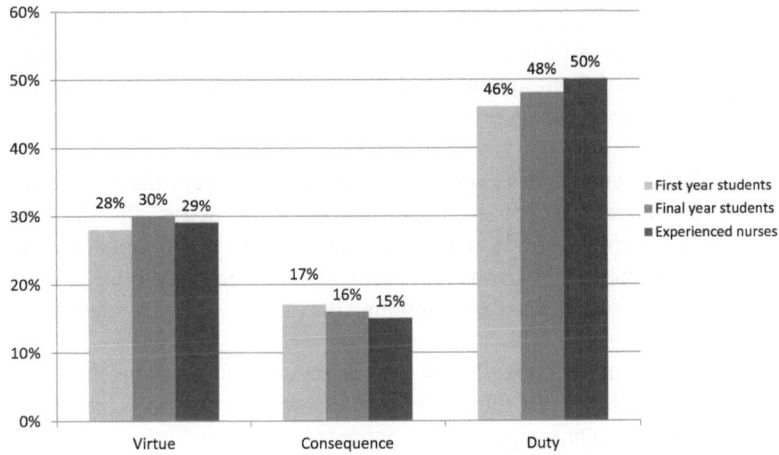

Chart 4.1 Reasons for Choosing Option 2 by Cohort (%)

that, at least for these respondents so far as Dilemma 1 was concerned, when clear rules or policies regarding how professionals should behave are available, direct appeal to such rules seems to be made in terms of justifying their choices. Here, it is perhaps worth raising a tentative suggestion drawn in relation to data derived from dilemmas used within the Jubilee Centre's *The Good Teacher* study that might be relevant here. This is that where the situation in the dilemmas involves colleague (broadly speaking where they concern whistleblowing) respondents seem to fall back on codes of conduct as a crutch to explain or justify their choice of action (Peterson and Arthur, 2020). Whether or not this is the case more generally, these findings serve as a reminder that duty-based reasons – including those that draw explicitly on professional codes of conduct – do form an important and legitimate part of moral decision-making processes. With specific regard to nurses, there may be an associated fear of blame or sanction within current regulatory and accountability systems.

Dilemma: friendly patient

In the next dilemma we consider here (Dilemma 6 in the original study), respondents were asked how they would respond to the following situation:

> You get on very well with Pat, a patient you have been looking after for a while. Pat has multiple health problems and is frequently admitted to hospital for management of exacerbations. You have discovered that you share an interest in environmental issues and that Pat has been running an online campaign to highlight the plight of Dolphins

being caught in fishing nets. This is a cause particularly close to your heart. Pat lives near to you and has suggested you meet up when Pat is discharged from hospital and that you exchange contact details and become Facebook friends. What would you do?

Respondents were given two options. Option 1 – accept the invitation or Option 2 – do not accept the invitation. As with each of the dilemmas, respondents were given six reasons for each of the two options and were asked to rank the three reasons that best matched their decision. For Option 1 – accept the invitation – the following six reasons were provided:

Reason 1: You get on well with Pat and care about the friendship.
Reason 2: Nothing in the professional code of conduct forbids getting involved in campaigns run by patients.
Reason 3: A just and caring person would take every opportunity to advance the cause.
Reason 4: This is an opportunity to do some good for a cause, which is close to your heart.
Reason 5: There is nothing wrong with making new friends.
Reason 6: You do not want to appear rude by refusing.

For Option 2 – do not accept the invitation – the following six reasons were provided:

Reason 1: It is generally imprudent to become friends with your patients.
Reason 2: Befriending patients is forbidden by professional codes of conduct.
Reason 3: It would be unfair to both you and Pat to begin a friendship you may later have to end for professional reasons.
Reason 4: You want to avoid trouble or criticism with your colleagues and employer.
Reason 5: You have a personal rule never to befriend your patients.
Reason 6: It could lead to problems if Pat is admitted in the future.

As with the first dilemma we considered earlier, there was a strong level of agreement between respondents about which option should be selected, with the majority (92.6%) selecting Option 2 – they would not accept the invitation. In contrast to the first dilemma, however, for this 92.6% of the respondents, *two* types of reasons were most commonly selected. As Chart 4.2 demonstrates, respondents placed little priority on consequence-based reasons and instead placed broadly comparable emphasis on virtue-based and duty-based reasons to explain their selection of Option 2. The

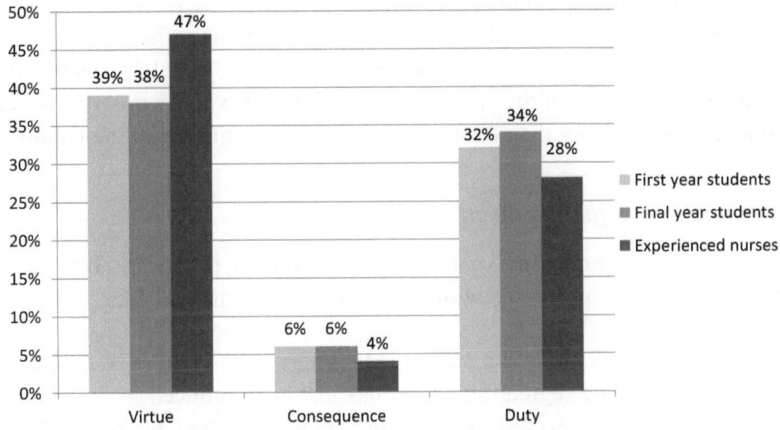

Chart 4.2 Reasons for Choosing Option 2 by Cohort (%)

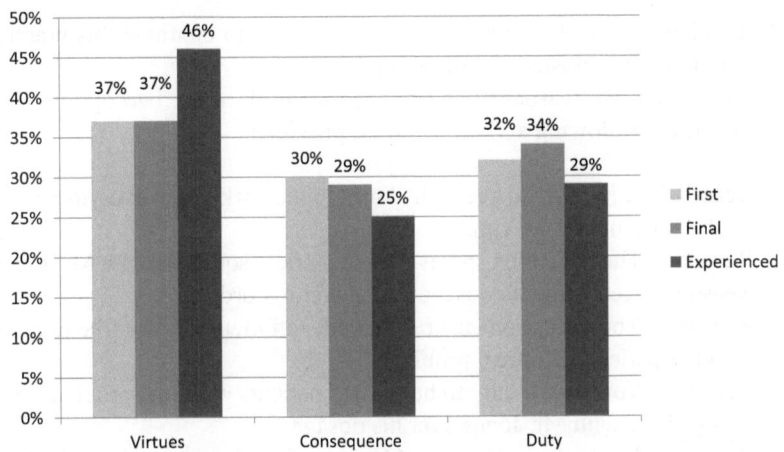

Chart 4.3 Overall Reasoning for Friendly Patient Dilemma Including Both Options 1 and 2 (%)

data also evidenced some similarities between respondents across the three career stages. Forty-seven per cent of experienced nurses, 39% of first-year undergraduate students and 38% of final-year undergraduate students selected virtue-based reasons (either that it is *imprudent* to become friends with patients or it is not *fair* on oneself or the patient to start a relationship). Thirty-two per cent of first-year undergraduate students, 34% of final-year undergraduate students and 28% of experienced nurses selected rule-based reasons (befriending patients is forbidden by professional codes of conduct and you have a personal rule of never to befriend your patients).

The interesting overall finding here, as shown in Chart 4.3, was that this is the only dilemma of the six used in the study for which virtue-based reasoning ranked higher than deontological reasoning among all the cohorts.

Dilemma: the difficult patient

In the third dilemma we examine here (dilemma 4 in the original study), respondents were presented with the following dilemma:

> It is the weekend and a patient, Mr. Jones, who is labelled 'difficult', is in pain. The regular analgesia has just been reduced in dose and so the volume is also reduced. The nurse prepares the new, reduced dose but makes the volume the same as the previous higher dose so that Mr. Jones cannot tell the difference. *What would you do?*

Respondents were offered two options. Option 1: to continue this practice and Option 2: to refuse to follow this practice.

Once again, six reasons were provided for each of the two options. For Option 1, the following six reasons were provided:

> Reason 1: It is wiser to keep Mr. Jones in the dark given everything else the staff must deal with.
> Reason 2: The deception spares you a pointless squabble with Mr. Jones.
> Reason 3: Reducing the dosage is the doctor's orders.
> Reason 4: The deception ensures that all staff members are free to assist other patients with real problems.
> Reason 5: You have a duty to help other patients with real problems, not squabble with Mr. Jones over his dosage.
> Reason 6: It is only kind to spare Mr. Jones from having to deal with both the pain and accept that he is not permitted a higher dose.

For Option 2, the following six reasons were provided:

> Reason 1: Trust between nurses and patients would be grievously damaged if nurses always deceived their patients like this.
> Reason 2: It is wrong to infantilise and manipulate patients like this.
> Reason 3: It is unwise to get into the habit of misleading people, even when it seems harmless.

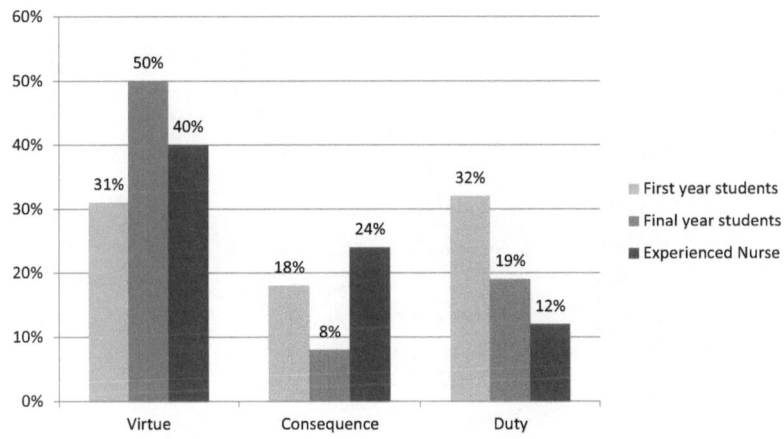

Chart 4.4 Reasons for Choosing Option 1 by Cohort (%)

Reason 4: You may get into trouble if your deception is discovered.
Reason 5: You want to be truthful to your patients about their care.
Reason 6: You are professionally obligated not to deceive your patients.

Though not at quite to the extent of the two dilemmas mentioned earlier, it is interesting to note that the dilemma constituted by the expert panel did not produce a significant divide in terms of the option selected. A total of 82.9% of respondents indicated that they would refuse to follow this practice (Option 2), with 17.1% reporting that they would follow this practice (Option 1). We now consider the reasons given for each option.

In selecting from the six reasons available for Option 1, 31% of first-year undergraduate students, 50% of final-year undergraduate students and 40% of the experienced nurses chose virtue-based reasons to explain their choice. Duty-based reasons for this option were chosen by 32% of first-year undergraduate students, 19% of final-year undergraduate students and 12% of experienced nurses (see Chart 4.4).

For Option 2, 37% of first-year undergraduate students, 33% of final-year undergraduate students and 32% of experienced nurses indicated that they would refuse to follow the practice for virtue-based reasons (as shown in Chart 4.5). Forty-one per cent of experienced nurses, 38% of final-year undergraduate students and 36% of first-year undergraduate students selected rule-based reasons (it is wrong to infantilise and manipulate patients like this or they are professionally obligated not to deceive

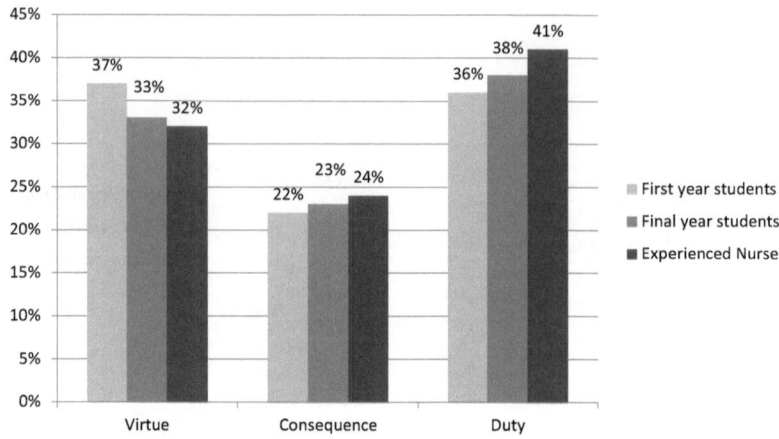

Chart 4.5 Reasons for Choosing Option 2 by Cohort (%)

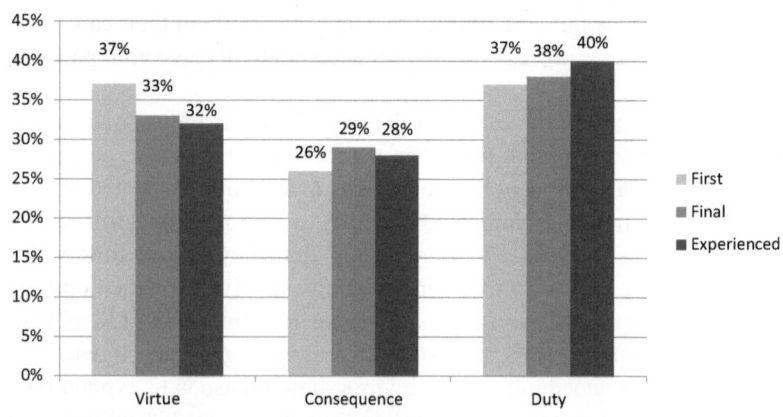

Chart 4.6 Overall Reasoning for Dilemma 4, Including Both Options 1 and 2 (%)

patients). As with the second dilemma considered earlier, the ranking of consequential reasons (trust between nurses and patients would be grievously damaged if nurses always deceived their patients like this or one may get into trouble if deception is discovered) was much lower than that of virtue- or duty-based reasons.

When we consider the reasons provided for both Options 1 and 2 and combine these for each cohort, and put together the three different reasoning

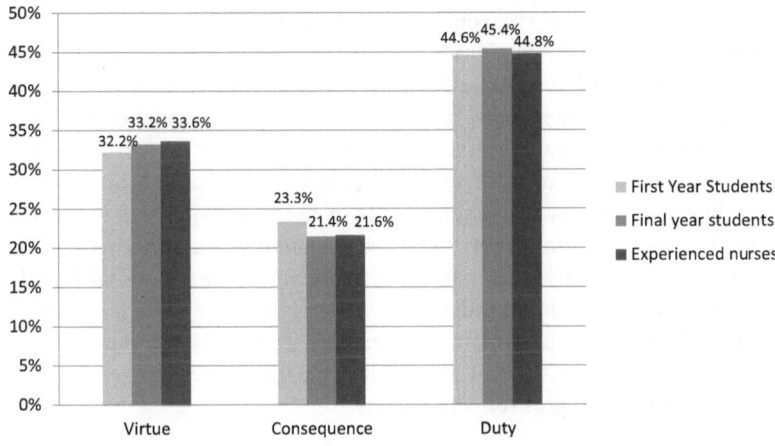

Chart 4.7 Overall Reasoning Across All Ethical Dilemmas (%)

modes (virtue based, duty based and consequentialist) in this scenario, 37% of first-year undergraduate students, 38% of final-year undergraduate students and 40% of experienced nurses opted for duty-based reasoning, as shown in Chart 4.6. The virtue-based reasoning percentages were only slightly lower, with 37% of first-year undergraduate students, 33% of final-year undergraduate students and 32% of experienced nurses opting for virtue-based reasons. These results suggest that for these respondents, duty-based and virtue-based reasons were given much greater attention than consequentialist reasons.

Looking across the dilemmas

In regard to the overall findings across the dilemmas, a clear finding of the study was that a majority of respondents across all career stages cited duty-based reasons as the motivation behind the options chosen: 44.6% of first-year students, 45.4% of final-year students and 44.8% of all experienced nurses. Though not to the level of duty-based reasons, virtue-based reasons also found notable expression in the choices selected by respondents, with 32.2% of first-year undergraduate students, 33.2% of final-year undergraduate students and 33.6% of experienced nurses citing these reasons. Considerations of consequences, however, ranked much lower than both duty-based and virtue-based reasoning, as can be seen from Chart 4.7.

The extent of duty-based reasoning was greater than in any of the professions studied by the Jubilee Centre for Character and Virtues. Important, too, is that reliance on duty-based reasoning, if anything, *increased* with experience. In most of the Centre's other studies on professional ethics, the results indicated that new entrants to the profession rely on virtue-based reasons, those at the end of their professional education cite rule-based reasons (in line with the formal requirements of the profession that students are being taught) and more experienced professionals return to virtue-based reasoning once they realise that many ethical dilemmas are uncodifiable and require a level of professional judgement. In the *Virtuous Practice in Nursing* study, however, this curve did not materialise from the data – duty-based reasons remained the most common at each of the three career stages. As the authors of the project report reflected, from

> the point of view of those theorists who consider virtue ethics the most appropriate moral paradigm for nursing, this is a worrying finding. There was no sign of virtue ethics having become the 'theory of choice' (Tschudin, 2010: 130) among nursing professionals.
>
> (Kristjánsson, Varghese *et al.*, 2017; for further analysis of this finding see Vargehese and Kristjánsson, 2018)

In the interviews, experienced nurses were asked about dilemmas they faced in their professional work. While respondents gave a number of examples of such dilemmas, there was no clear and unified sense across the experienced nurses of how they sought to deal with situations in which dilemmas arise. Some respondents spoke of a distinction between personal commitments (what respondents generally referred to as 'values') and their professional conduct and suggested that these personal commitments were private and did not/should not impact on their approach with patients (examples here included religious commitments and situations in which choices made by patients and families differed from those they would make themselves as a patient or parent). The interview data suggested that the experienced nurses generally developed their own stances when faced with dilemmas. Only a few mentioned the importance of professional judgement, with more stating that they are always guided by a sense of what is best for the patients. Very little reference was made to professional codes in guiding conduct. These latter two findings are interesting given the survey data presented earlier and the importance we have attached to professional judgement in earlier chapters. Yet, there were some other interesting insights – which again speak to context and professional development – that can also be gleaned from the interview data.

The first is the impact of time and role on the ability to practice professional judgement. Some respondents suggested that this became easier with experience and seniority, suggesting through either personal reflection or in general terms that an experienced nurse would find it easier to exercise their professional judgement. One experienced nurse spoke of the challenges faced by new nurses who could find it difficult to practice their professional conduct given the reality of healthcare provision. This nurse concluded: *'their values – what they would do as a nurse, their gold standard, they're not able to do'*. Another nurse spoke of her own experiences and recounted situations in which a patient wished to know that they were dying but the relatives did not want them to be told. The nurse affirmed:

> that is really, really hard, because it's very clear that you should tell them, but it's very difficult to be the one person that will stand up against the [family]. And I had a very similar situation to that in the hospital, when I was newly qualified that they didn't want us to tell them, and I didn't. There's no way I was going up against matron to do that at that point. Ten years down the line and I would.

In these words, we get a clear sense that as this nurse has become more experienced, practiced and confident in their judgement, a different course of action would be chosen.

The second insight, which on the surface may seem like something of a contradiction, was that rather than making it easier to exercise professional judgement, experience and seniority can lead to a reduction of the space and flexibility required. Here, some of the experienced nurses mentioned how the 'system' worked against professional freedom and conduct as captured in the following extract:

> The higher up you go, the harder it is to be that person because you will get sucked into a system that's trying to perform in ways that it's not possible any more. We're governed by a government that wants targets, and nobody will stand up and say we can't meet them. So it is quite tough, to be a compassionate, caring person, in certain roles.

Learning professional ethics

In light of the aforementioned findings, and to add further depth to our analysis, we turn now to questions about the learning of professional ethics by nurses. In order to do so, we draw on two sources of data from the *Virtuous Practice in Nursing* study – interviews with experienced nurses and interviews with a small selection of nursing educators. As we examined in

Chapter 2, the extant literature on nursing education and professional ethics recognises that learning to become a nurse has an important moral dimension in addition (and indeed not necessarily unrelated) to the knowledge and skills modern nurses require. While recognising the limitations of the sample size involved, analysis of the interview data raises some noteworthy themes.

The first of these themes is the mixed picture that the experienced nurses presented of their preparation as nurses. A number of the experienced nurses reported that, in retrospect, they believed that they had been underprepared for the pressures of enacting professionalism in practice. The following experienced nurse suggested that:

> I don't think it prepared you at all, really. I think being at university is so different to working on a ward. I think also, while you are at university, you get told to think in a certain way, and obviously, if you have alternative views, then that is frowned upon and you are always worried that you are going to get into trouble. So, I think, even though the university gives you the background, and the placements to enable you to interact with patients, I think, really I don't think it is the university profession, I think it is a type of profession that you should learn on the job.

Another experienced nurse raised a similar point, adding that patients themselves could play a key role in this educational process in terms of helping beginning nurses to understand patient-centred care:

> I think nurses a lot more need to be encouraged to sort of put themselves into patients' shoes really. And spend more time actually listening to patients in their training, whether you get patients in, I don't know what form this training takes, these days, maybe this already happens. But I think one of the greatest educators to us is patients themselves. And explaining what they want from us, and how they want it, and we need to be listening to that.

The view expressed here that speaks to the 'golden rule' of nursing (Corazzini *et al.*, 2005) – that is, treating the patient as nurses themselves would wish to be treated or they would wish a close relative of theirs to be treated – came through in interviews with other experienced nurses. One of the experienced nurses spoke at some length about the need for educational processes and activities that enabled nursing students to come together collaboratively to engage in reflective dialogue about their actual experiences:

> But I think if we encouraged students on placement to come back with a reflective piece about an ethical dilemma that they could then debate

and discuss in the class, it links it to real people and they'd have to be confidential when they're coming back with a piece, but sometimes, particularly when it's younger students, they're not life experienced and they can't always imagine what would they do if . . . They need to see it and feel it and believe it, come back and reflect on it. So it would need to be a joint placement and theory thing. But linking that with a real person that they've been in contact with.

Another experienced nurse also pointed to the value of collaborative reflective dialogue in the context of their own concerns about the education of nurses, also referencing their apprehension about the move to nursing being a graduate entry profession:

I'm quite direct in my view about that really. I think that the move away from schools of nursing and into universities has been the death of the nursing profession. I really strongly believe that we are trying to be all things to all people and achieving none of those things now. I meet students that come onto the wards that have no idea what being a nurse is about, none whatsoever and I am very clear that, you know, I had six weeks induction, in my six weeks in school, preparing for your first placement and then you are out on the wards. I learnt how to be a nurse and how not to be a nurse by the people that I worked with and you came back into the School of Nursing and then you discussed and you reflected and you talked and you had an opportunity to think about and evaluate what you'd done and I don't suppose in those days I really knew what it was I was, I couldn't articulate it like that, but I knew what was good and what wasn't good and I knew what I wanted to be and what I didn't want to be. I really do believe that the current training is not fit for purpose and doesn't prepare nurses that are able to be nurses.

To provide one further point on this first theme, some of the experienced nurses connected the lack of time spent developing professional practice based around care and compassion with more structural issues facing nursing education and nursing more generally:

Unfortunately I think students don't tend to spend a lot of time with senior staff, so they tend to spend most of their time with low graded staff who are there doing the very basic nursing tasks. And they haven't always got those, that confidence and the different strengths and traits that you perhaps want to see flourishing in nurses. I think one of the things that would be really valuable is about nurses spending more time with staff who are of a more senior level, to see how things operate and to also have an understanding of organisations as a whole. I think sometimes when you work in particular area or one ward, it becomes very easy to just see what's happening in your area and you'll say, 'We've got no staff today,' or something like that or, 'We've got all these patients today'. Whereas actually it's about what's going on in the whole organisation, how things slot together and fit together.

(Experienced Nurse)

In light of these criticisms of the learning of professional ethics, it is interesting to consider how these more critical views correlate with those of the nursing educators and final-year undergraduate students interviewed in the study. Not surprisingly, the nursing educators were more positive about their role and practice in relation to educating professional ethics, typically placing reflection, and indeed providing an informed and critical space for such reflection, as central to their work. One nursing educator shared their view of the importance of supporting their nursing students to bring together various factors in order to critically examine their burgeoning sense of professional ethics and practice:

You always teach people to reflect, and you always teach people to reflect on what have I seen in clinical practice, what have I seen in my personal life – and what's the connection between the two? Because you can present someone with a medical diagnosis, but it how it impacts on them, how it impacts on patients, how it impacts on people's functionality; and that's the material you want students to engage with. Take the theory that they're taught the classroom and marry it with material that they see on placement; sort of the lived experience components of the course. And, as I said, a large part of it is also thinking the correlation [with] what happens in their personal lives as well.

(Nursing Educator)

Cognisant of the challenges facing nursing educators, and of resonance given the concerns about the professional education of nurses raised by the experienced nurses, one of the nursing educators spoke at some length about the barriers they faced in engaging with professional ethics on nursing programmes and how they desired to do more.

so there are certain virtues that more readily align themselves to professional nursing issues and communication, for example. We could teach much more about that but we don't because like all curriculum within the healthcare arena, it tends to get dominated by the scientific, task oriented must-do's and the curriculum. I've had experience of how that's done differently in different courses and also with having had some involvement in teaching in other programs, including medical education in the past, I think nursing actually is way behind in that regard. There's pastoral groups and debriefing groups and restorative supervision and peer supervision models in most other healthcare curricula and I don't understand really why that isn't prioritised in nursing, particularly when nursing has led the way with models around reflective practice and reflective practice, yet we seem to have gone backwards from that point with actually demonstrating how to do it well. I guess I'm still not answering your question about what we teach in relation to values.

(Nursing Educator)

Interestingly, the final-year undergraduate students gave different accounts of the extent of engagement with ethical aspects of nursing on their courses. While all reported that ethical dimensions of nursing were present within their university courses, only a few held the view that their time at university had prepared them well in this regard. More commonly, the final-year undergraduate students suggested that they would have welcomed more attention to ethics in their programmes, including greater cohesiveness between university-based sessions and their practical placement experiences. This was often framed in terms of both university sessions needing to do more to bring ethical dilemmas encountered on placements into consideration with tutors and fellow students and a need to focus the ethical on being patient centred.

To conclude this first theme, these responses present a picture that may present room for concern, though we must, of course, note the restrictions of the sample. What they do suggest is the importance of careful and intentional planning for how professional ethics are encountered by nursing students – including in ways that connect theoretical and more detached principles and ideas with engaged, actual practices and experiences.

A second, and not unrelated, theme of interest relating to learning professional ethics that came out of the interview data with experienced nurses and nursing educators is the importance placed by the former on role models, with a number stating how they had learned from the craft and wisdom of colleagues in applied situations. One experienced nurse, for instance, stated that 'learning your nursing skills from role models on the ward was the main' formative process in their professional development, implicitly emphasising the collaborative, supportive and reflective environment needed to cultivate professional wisdom. The following experienced nurse also emphasised the educational value of role models, while also highlighting that the modelling of poor conduct by others can also impact on beginning nurses:

> What helped? I think a good role model is always good to have. I had good role models and I could still identify – because I did start as an auxiliary as well, before I did my training – and even then I identified . . . There was a nurse who was . . . I think she was an acting sister or something, she was my role model – she was very caring, compassionate. You could see that she had the personal bit and she was very helpful to relatives, and I remember looking at her thinking, 'That's the kind of nurse I want to be.' You heard less tolerant nurses and you thought, 'That's not the kind of nurse I want to be.' I suppose that does shape your behaviours, both the positive and the less positive.

The importance of learning from positive role models was also mentioned by several of the nursing educators interviewed, reflecting a core theme in the virtue-focused literature surveyed in Chapter 2 (see, e.g., Vanlaere and Gastmans, 2007), though this was not so clearly and comprehensively seen across the nursing educator interviews to the extent found in those with the experienced nurses. In instances where the importance of learning from role models was mentioned, these were connected with reflective assignments and other university-led tasks or – as in the following examples – remained either at a general, rather than precise, level or was something the nurse educator themselves aimed to be:

> Students will very often come back from practice and say, 'My mentor was brilliant, she was really good. That's the kind of nurse I want to be.' Or they'll come back and say, 'I saw nurses out there, and that's not the nurse, the kind of nurse I want to be.' So I think the role modelling with relation to practice has got a big influence for us working in education.
>
> (Nurse Educator)

> I think you have to demonstrate, like the role modelling as well and however frustrated sometimes I get with the students, I always, with the first years, I do try and show them support and I think that classroom behaviour and listening and respect is really important and the encouragement, when people come up with their ideas and sharing as well.
>
> (Nurse Educator)

What did not come through to the extent we might expect, was detailed exposition of the importance of nursing students reflecting on their care practices as a fully intentional and integrated aspect of programmes. It would seem that the questions about the depth and consistency of ethics education in nursing programmes cited in Chapter 2 remain relevant.

A third theme of interest deriving from the interview data with experienced nurses and nursing educators concerned their relationship with the NMC Code. While all of the nursing educators attested to the importance of the Code, two patterns of usage were reported. Some of the nursing educators stated that the Code formed the central plank of learning professional ethics for their students, as in the following instance:

It's [the Code] the main basis. Whenever you're talking about nursing practice, you have to ensure that what you're teaching is reflective of the code. So for example, in terms of expectations of the nurse then that has to be conveyed to the student and it generally comes along in terms of safe practice, ethical practice, areas like that.

Another made clear that students on their programme 'absolutely have a degree of accountability to the code – and they're very well aware of that'. While in no way suggesting that the Code is unimportant, a second form of positioning of the Code was reported by other nursing educators. This represented the Code as being important but less dominant in day-to-day care. One nursing educator captured this by stating their view that the Code acts as 'a guide. It's a guide for me, it's a guide to the students', while another referred to the Code as 'a fallback position, that if you break the code of conduct, then we've got something to fall back on'. This latter nursing educator continued that they while they 'occasionally make reference to it. I don't think I've ever once given a stand-up lecture solely about the code of conduct, but it's the kind of thing you frequently drop into lectures'. Aligned with these views was the idea that sitting alongside and within the Code were an enduring set of qualities that give shape to professional ethics and identity, as captured by the following nursing educator: 'I go back to the key things of that I was taught, which haven't really changed. So, beneficence, non-beneficence, confidentiality, the consent, to whether a trusting relationships, [and] having a level of humility'. Similarly, another nursing educator stated that:

I've been nursing since 1985. So for me the NMC code is . . . It's just there. It's part of me. I don't really ever look at it, I don't think about it because I know that I don't accept gifts from patients. It's about being non-judgemental. It's about communicating, working effectively as part of a team. Because that's just what my practice has always been. So I've not really ever had to check anything on the code, because, I just haven't.

It was this latter view of the Code – as providing a foundation without capturing professional ethics in full – that was expressed more commonly by the experienced nurses in the study. One experienced nurse explained that the 'NMC provide a good foundation for the minimum requirement' and that 'it would be impossible to capture the more intangible elements and the variety in some of the great nurses that are in the service'. Another spoke of how the Code represented 'something that is there, at the back of your mind' but continued:

> It is very difficult to say whether it matches up to what being a good nurse is about. I mean it has changed, since I have qualified, and I think there needs to be more about kindness in there. I feel like I already have the virtues in place that make me a good nurse, without having to worry about the code of practice. I feel like honesty is one of the most important characteristics of being a nurse. You know, so patients can trust you.

Other experienced nurses conveyed very similar messages, speaking of the engaged nature of professional ethics in practice. In the final extract we share, a real sense given that the Code fails to capture the essence of what it means to be a nurse and that this had been 'moved so far away from that, that actually that message is lost':

> the single most important message when I qualified, was you are the patient's advocate, you must do the right thing for them and you must speak up for them and do the thing that is right for them, even if it's not what the doctor wants you to do . . . I think the Code of Conduct should be that. It should be your sword and your shield, it should be your, look, I cannot do that, I cannot do what you're asking me to do because it's against my professional Code of Conduct

Once again here we have the focus on the patient, and caring for the needs of the patient, as the touchstone of a nurse's ethical practice.

Conclusion

In this chapter, we have presented and analysed data to provide insights into how nurses at different stages of their career responded to a set of ethical dilemmas. While any data obtained in relation to abstract, though applied, dilemmas come with important caveats, drawing on the analysis of the original study – and extending this with our own subsequent analysis – we can see how the respondents in the study prioritised duty-based reasons over consequentialist and virtue-based reasons. In the second, the majority of the respondents identified virtue-based reasons as their motivation to choose their preferred options, while in the third, a conflict was found between duty-based and virtue-based reasoning among the respondents. Perhaps more significantly, when we look across the dilemma data, it is clear that the majority of respondents across the three career stages cited duty-based reasons as the motivation behind the options chosen, with virtue-based reasons also finding notable expression in the choices selected. In contrast, considerations of consequences were selected to a much lower degree than both duty-based and virtue-based reasonings. As we have reflected here (see also Arthur *et al.*, 2019a; Varghese and Kristjánsson, 2018), the extent of duty-based reasoning was greater than that found in studies conducted by the Jubilee Centre. Moreover, this recourse to duty-based reasoning, if anything, *increased* with experience.

We have also drawn upon interview data with experienced nurses and nursing educators to examine their perceptions of how nurses are prepared for the ethical dimensions of their work. These interviews suggest that while some respondents place the NMC Code as core to their practice, most experienced nurses and nurse educators interviewed understand the Code as being a fall back and/or as crutch to rely on. On this latter view, these experienced nurses and nurse educators place more importance on core professional virtues, such as care, compassion, honesty and beneficence, viewing these are of greater importance in their daily professional lives. Oftentimes, these qualities were spoken of alongside – and indeed as integral to – the golden rule of nursing; that is, giving patients the level of care a nurse would want for themselves and their families. Associated too with this sentiment and commitment was a sense that, for at least some of these respondents, a 'good' nurse is one who acts as an advocate for their patients. The interview data, too, present a varied picture of nurses' education so far as professional ethics are concerned. While role modelling, reflection and collaborative discussion about professional dilemmas were all raised as playing a key role in such learning, a number of the experienced nurses expressed that they had not felt prepared for the ethical dimensions of their professional practice, raising further questions about the educational processes necessary for being a good nurse (see Honkavuo, 2021 for an interesting account of ethics simulation in nursing education). In light of these findings, and those presented in the previous chapter, we move now to provide some overall conclusions and recommendations.

Note

1   For more regarding the design of the situational judgement tests, see www.jubileecentre.ac.uk/professions

Conclusions, recommendations and further research

Introduction

Nursing as a profession is inherently concerned with virtues and virtuous actions. As others have suggested, and as we have contended throughout this book, the nursing profession and the nurses that comprise it are guided by notions of care, compassion and kindness. Yet, it must not be assumed that all nurses conceive these virtues in identical ways, nor that nurses all rely equally on their character when faced with challenging ethical situations in their practice. Moreover, nurses learn and work in complex healthcare settings, some aspects of which support virtuous practice and some aspects of which constrain the levels and form of care patients receive. Hence, this requires forms of nursing education and professional development that embrace the complexities of professional practice and that bring nurses together to consider the guidelines that govern their practice (including the NMC Code) and to engage in shared dialogue and reflection about the ethical aspects of their work – including those aspects that defy simple solutions.

In the last two chapters, we have presented and analysed a range of empirical data to present a picture of how nurses at various stages of their career, as well as nursing educators, conceive the ethical nature of their professional role – including the character strengths they identify as being central to nursing. In this final chapter, we set out in short form the overall findings, before offering some recommendations based on the preceding analysis. Finally, we advance several areas that would benefit from further research.

Overall findings

The findings stemming from the *Virtuous Practice in Nursing* study and the additional analysis given in these pages can be summarised as

DOI: 10.4324/9781003146308-6

follows (see also Kristjánsson, Varghese *et al.*, 2017 and Thompson *et al.*, 2021):

- The nurses in this study appreciated the ethical dimensions of their work, viewing themselves as advocates for their patients and presenting nursing as concerned with virtues such as compassion, care, honesty and kindness.
- The notion of caring for others played an important role in the reported motivations for entering the profession. This motivation is often connected to the care received by nurses in earlier life or by that received by a close relative or friend.
- Nurses across the three career stages were in substantial agreement on the virtues that 'good' nurses should possess:

  - Kindness
  - Honesty
  - Teamwork

- While the experienced nurses in the study spoke positively of the levels of professional autonomy they enjoyed in their workplaces, they also expressed serious concerns about the significant challenges faced in terms of being the sort of nurse they desired. These challenges included: staff shortages, pressures on time and limited resources.
- Amidst these significant challenges, experienced nurses identified a supportive, collaborative workplace environment and the influence of positive role models as of particular importance in enabling and sustaining their ability to live out their character as nurses.
- When faced with ethical dilemmas, the nurses at different career stages demonstrated an ability to integrate moral reasoning into their practice and to draw on a range of considerations to reflect upon and adjudicate ethical issues. Regarding responses to the survey data, an unusual picture emerged with respect to other Jubilee Centre reports on professional ethics: namely, the absence of a U-curve where virtue-based reasoning picks up steadily with experience after a dip during years of formal education. In this study, little change was observed from one cohort to another, and duty-based modes of reasoning remain the most common ones across the three career stages in the study.
- Experienced nurses and nursing educators reported a variety of thoughts regarding how nursing ethics is approached within the curriculums of nursing schools. Some nursing educators placed the NMC Code as central to the ethical aspects of students' learning, while others identified more of a background or implicit role for the Code. While nursing

educators largely agreed about the importance of attending to the ethical dimensions of nursing, the accounts of both final-year undergraduates and experienced nurses suggest that more attention to dialogue, reflection and role modelling is needed on nursing education programmes.

Overall recommendations

Having presented these overall findings, we now move to draw on and extend on the recommendations contained within the original project report (Kristjánsson, Varghese *et al.*, 2017) to propose the following overall recommendations:

- More explicit attention to character and virtue needs to be included in the curriculum for preparing nurses. This effort should help student nurses to consider real-life ethical dimensions of their work through collaborative dialogue with others, through reflection and through learning with and from role models. The idea of patient-centred practice, including the nurse as advocate for patients, should be front and centre of this explicit attention.
- As stated earlier, role modelling is a crucial formative process in developing character. As such, it should be placed at the very heart of nursing education, with nursing students interacting with and learning from those experienced nurses whose conduct is commensurate with compassionate, patient-centred care.
- While role modelling is critical, nurses at all stages of their careers need intentional and ongoing opportunities to understand and reflect upon the ethical dimensions of their work. This includes the time and space to come together (e.g., in small groups) to discuss real-life ethical quandaries and the potential responses. Such time, space and opportunities are particularly crucial for nurses at all stages of their careers and may help to counterbalance the obvious and very real challenges that nurses face in enacting their professional characters.

Future research

The analysis of data presented in this book highlights a number of possible directions for future research. To extend current understandings of what constitutes 'the good nurse', including the educational processes involved, the following are particularly relevant:

- Noting the publication of the Nursing and Midwifery Council's Standards for education and training in 2019, further research examining and assessing the impact on professional ethics in nursing programmes would be timely – including whether the standards have increased the amount of attention given to nursing ethics and, if so, how this has been formulated within programmes. Of particular relevance and interest is to know more about the role a positive learning culture attentive to professional ethics can play a vital part in empowering nursing students in their professional character.

- Given its importance to a virtue ethics approach to professional ethics, further research is needed that examines the professional wisdom of nurses, including how this wisdom is mediated, negotiated and enacted in practice.
- As the data suggest the absence of a U-curve in the types of reasons given in regard to the ethical dilemmas (namely, the absence of a U-curve where virtue-based reasoning picks up steadily with experience after a dip during years of formal education), more research is needed to understand whether this is replicated with other cohorts of respondents and, if so, that interrogates in more detail the reasons for this absence.
- While the study reported here sought the views of respondents across three points in a nursing career (first-year undergraduate, final-year undergraduate and nurses with five years or more experience), longitudinal research tracking the same nurse(s) over a sustained period of time is likely to obtain a deeper sense of the trajectories and nuances of the ethical dimensions of nursing in practice. Looking more specifically at *phronesis*, longitudinal studies would enable insight into how this meta-virtue is developed throughout a nurse's career. Furthermore, longitudinal studies would provide an apt way to understand more about both moral distress and also the relation between non-moral character strengths (such as resilience) and the moral character of nurses.
- As with other books in this series (Peterson and Arthur, 2020; Jameel *et al.*, 2021), we would also suggest that the interplay between developing the virtues and the role/impact of organisational culture needs further exploration. It is clear from this research that work environments and educational institutions have an impact on virtues in context. Organisations and institutions need to realise the importance of orchestrating the climate that enables clinicians to flourish, and we need to know more about how this can and does occur.

References

Adams, P. (2009) 'Ethics with character: Virtues and the ethical social worker', *The Journal of Sociology & Social Welfare*. 36 (3). 83–105.

Ahlstedt, C., Eriksson Lindvall, C., Holmström, I. K. and Muntlin, Å. (2020) 'Flourishing at work: Nurses' motivation through daily communication – An ethnographic approach', *Nursing & Health Sciences*. 22 (4). 1169–1176.

Armstrong, A. E. (2006) 'Towards a strong virtue ethics for nursing practice', *Nursing Philosophy*. 7 (3). 110–124.

Armstrong, A. E. (2007) *Nursing Ethics: A Virtue-Based Approach*. Basingstoke: Palgrave Macmillan.

Armstrong, A. E., Parsons, S. and Barker, P. J. (2000) 'An inquiry into moral virtues, especially compassion, in psychiatric nursing: Findings from a Delphi study', *Journal of Psychiatric and Mental Health Nursing*. 7. 297–306.

Arthur, J. and Earl, S. R. (2020) *Character in the Professions: How Virtue Informs Professional Practice*. Birmingham: Jubilee Centre for Character and Virtues, University of Birmingham.

Arthur, J., Earl, S. R., Thompson, A. P. and Ward, J. W. (2019a) *Repurposing the Professions: The Role of Professional Character – Initial Insights*. Birmingham: Jubilee Centre for Character and Virtues.

Arthur, J., Earl, S. R., Thompson, A. P. and Ward, J. W. (2019b) 'The value of character-based judgement in the professional domain', *Journal of Business Ethics*. DOI: 10.1007/s10551-019-04269-7.

Arthur, J., Kristjánsson, K., Cooke, S., Brown, E. and Carr, D. (2015) *The Good Teacher: Understanding Virtues in Practice*. Birmingham: Jubilee Centre for Character and Virtues.

Arthur, J., Kristjánsson, K., Thomas, H., Holdsworth, M., Badini Confolonieri, L. and Qiu, T. (2014) *Virtuous Character for the Practice of Law: Research Report*. Birmingham: Jubilee Centre for Character and Virtues, University of Birmingham.

Arthur, J., Kristjánsson, K., Thomas, H., Kotzee, B., Ignatowicz, A. and Qiu, T. (2015) *Virtuous Medical Practice*. Birmingham: Jubilee Centre for Character and Virtues.

Arthur, J., Walker, D. I. and Thoma, S. J. (2018) *Soldiers of Character: Research Report*. Birmingham: Jubilee Centre for Character and Virtues, University of Birmingham.

Banks, S. and Gallagher, A. (2009) *Ethics in Professional Life: Virtues for Health and Social Care*. London: Red Globe Press.

Bessant, J. (2009) 'Aristotle meets youth work: A case for virtue ethics', *Journal of Youth Studies*. 12 (4). 423–438.

Bishop, A. H. and Scudder, J. R. (1996) *Nursing Ethics: Therapeutic Caring Presence*. Sudbury, MA: Jones and Bartlett.

Blond, P., Antonacopoulou, E. and Pabst, A. (2015) *In Professions We Trust: Fostering Virtuous Practitioners in Teaching, Law and Medicine*. London: Respublica.

Bohlin, K. (2005) *Teaching Character Education Through Literature: Awakening the Moral Imagination in Secondary Classrooms*. London: Routledge.

Bontemps-Hommen, C. M. M. L., Baart, A. and Vosman, F. T. H. (2019) 'Practical wisdom in complex medical practices: A critical proposal', *Medicine, Health-Care and Philosophy*. 22. 95–105.

Brody, H. and Doukas, D. (2014) 'Professionalism: A framework to guide medical education', *Medical Education*. 48 (10). 980–987.

Campbell, A. V. and Chin, J. J. (2011) 'Preserving medical ethics and professionalism: Meeting the challenges of modern practice', *Annals Academy of Medicine Singapore*. 40 (1). 1–3.

Carr, D. (1999) 'Professional education and professional ethics', *Journal of Applied Philosophy*. 16 (1). 33–46.

Carr, D. (2011) 'Virtue, character and emotion in people professions: Towards a virtue ethics of interpersonal professional conduct', in L. Bondi, D. Carr, C. Clark, and C. Clegg (eds.) *Towards Professional Wisdom: Practical Deliberation in the People Professions*. Farnham: Ashgate.

Carr, D. (2018) 'Introduction', in D. Carr (ed.) *Cultivating Moral Character and Virtue in Professional Practice*. Abingdon: Routledge, pp. 1–12.

Cooke, S. and Carr, D. (2014) 'Virtue, practical wisdom and character in teaching', *British Journal of Educational Studies*. 62 (2). 91–110.

Corazzini, K. N., Lekan-Rutledge, D., Utley-Smith, Q., Piven, M. L., Colon-Emeric, C. S., Bailey, D., Ammarell, N. and Anderson, R. A. (2005) ' "The golden rule": Only a starting point for quality care', *Director*. 14 (1). 255–293.

Corley, M. C. (2002) 'Nurse moral distress: A proposed theory and research agenda', *Nursing Ethics*. 9 (6). 636–650.

Dixon-Woods, M., Yeung, K. and Bosk, C.L. (2011) 'Why is UK medicine No Longer a Self-Regulating Profession? The role of scandals involving "bad apple" doctors', *Social Science & Medicine*. 73 (10). 1452–1459.

Edmonson, C. (2010) 'Moral courage and the nurse leader', *OJIN: The Online Journal of Issues in Nursing*. 15 (3). Manuscript 5.

Eurofound (2012) *European Quality of Life Survey 2012*. Dublin: Eurofound. www.eurofound.europa.eu/sites/default/files/ef_publication/field_ef_document/ef1264en_0.pdf; accessed 1 May 2021.

Fish, D. and de Cossart, L. (2013) *Reflection for Medical Appraisal: Exploring and Developing Your Clinical Expertise and Professional Identity*. Gloucester: Aneumi Publications.

Flynn, M. and Mercer, D. (2013) 'Is compassion possible in a market-led NHS?' *Nursing Times*. 109 (7). 12–14.

Foth, T. and Holmes, D. (2016) 'Neoliberalism and the government of nursing through competency-based education', *Nursing Inquiry*. DOI: 10.1111/nin.12154.

Fourie, C. (2015) 'Moral distress and moral conflict in clinical ethics', *Bioethics*. 29 (2). 91–97.

Furlong, W., Crossan, M., Gandz, J. and Crossan, I. (2017) 'Character's essential role in addressing misconduct in financial institutions', *Business Law International*. 18. 199.

Gallagher, A. (2020) *Slow Ethics and the Art of Care*. Bingley: Emerald Press.

Gastmans, C., Dierckx de Casterlé, B. and Schotsmans, P. (1998) 'Nursing considered as moral practice: A philosophical – ethical interpretation of nursing', *Kennedy Institute of Ethics Journal*. 8. 43–69.

George, M. (2017) 'The effect of introducing new public management practices on compassion within the NHS', *Nursing Times*. 113 (7). 30–34.

Gillies, J. (2005) 'Getting it right in the consultation: Hippocrates's problems, Aristotle's solution', Occasional Paper 86. RGCP.

Gilligan, C. (1982) *In a Different Voice*. Cambridge: Harvard University Press.

Glaser, B. and Strauss, A. (1967) *The Discovery of Grounded Theory*. Hawthorne, NY: Aldine Publishing Company.

Grady, C., Danis, M., Soeken, K. L., O'Donnell, P., Taylor, C., Farrar, A. and Ulrich, C. M. (2008) 'Does ethics education influence the moral action of practicing nurses and social workers?' *The American Journal of Bioethics*. 8 (4). 4–11.

Great Britain. Parliament. House of Commons (2013) *Report of the Mid Staffordshire NHS Foundation Trust Public Inquiry by Francis, R*. London: The Stationary Office (HC 2012–2013 898–1).

Haggerty, L. and Grace, P. (2008) 'Clinical wisdom: The essential foundation of "good" nursing care', *Journal of Professional Nursing*. 16 (4). 404–408.

Harrison, T. and Khatoon, B. (2017) *Virtue, Practical Wisdom and Professional Education: A Pilot Intervention Designed to Enhance Virtue Knowledge, Understanding and Reasoning in Student Lawyers, Doctors and Teachers*. Birmingham: Jubilee Centre for Character and Virtues.

Holbeche, L. and Springett, N. (2004) *In Search of Meaning at Work*. Horsham: Roffey Park Institute. http://citeseerx.ist.psu.edu/viewdoc/download?doi=10.1.1.458.1538&rep=rep1&type=pdf; accessed 18 May 2018.

Holland, S. (2010) 'Scepticism about the virtue ethics approach to nursing ethics', *Nursing Philosophy*. 11 (3). 151–158.

Honkavuo, L. (2021) 'Ethics simulation in nursing education: Nursing students' experiences', *Nursing Ethics*. 1–13. DOI: 10.1177/0969733021994188.

Hoskins, K., Grady, C. and Ulrich, C. M. (2018) 'Ethics education in nursing: Instruction for future generation of nurses', *OJIN: The Online Journal of Issues in Nursing*. 23 (1). Manuscript 3.

The Independent (2013) 'The Francis report: The key findings', www.independent.co.uk/life-style/health-and-families/health-news/francis-report-key-findings-8484071.html; accessed 2 April 2021.

Ipsos MORI (2019) 'Ipsos MORI veracity index 2019: Trust in the professions survey', www.ipsos.com/sites/default/files/ct/news/documents/2019-11/trust-in-professions-veracity-index-2019-slides.pdf; accessed 21 May 2021.

Jameel, S., Peterson, A. and Arthur, J. (2021) *Ethics and the Good Doctor: Character in the Professional Domain*. Abingdon: Routledge.

Jameton, A. (1984) *Nursing Practice: The Ethical Issues*. Englewood Cliffs, NJ: Prentice Hall.

Jenkins, K., Kinsella, E. A. and DeLuca, S. (2019) 'Perspectives on phronesis in professional nursing practice', *Nursing Philosophy*. 20 (1). https://doi.org/10.1111/nup.12231.

Kalisch, B. J., Lee, H. and Rochman, M. (2010) 'Nursing staff teamwork and job satisfaction', *Journal of Nursing Management*. 18 (8). 938–947.

Kelly, B. (1993) 'The "real world" of hospital nursing practice as perceived by nursing undergraduates', *Journal of Professional Nursing*. 9. 27–33.

Kim, K., Han, Y. and Kim, J. (2015) 'Korean nurses' ethical dilemmas, professional values and professional quality of life', *Nursing Ethics*. 22 (4). 467–478.

Kinsella, E. A. and Pitman, A. (2012) 'Engaging phronesis in professional practice and education', in E. A. Kinsella and A. Pitman (eds.) *Phronesis as Professional Knowledge: Practical Wisdom in the Professions*. Dordecht: Sense Publishers, pp. 1–11.

Ko, H.-K., Tseng, H.-C., Chin, C.-C. and Hsu, M.-T. (2020) 'Phronesis of nurses: A response to moral distress', *Nursing Ethics*. 27 (1). 67–76.

Kotzee, B., Paton, A. and Conroy, M. (2016) 'Towards an empirically informed account of *phronesis* in medicine', *Perspectives in Biology and Medicine*. 59 (3). 337–350.

Krautscheid, L. and Brown, M. (2014) 'Microethical decision making among baccalaureate nursing students: A qualitative investigation', *The Journal of Nursing Education*. 53 (3). 19.

Kristjánsson, K. (2015a) 'Phronesis as an ideal in professional medical ethics: Some preliminary positionings and problematics', *Theoretical Medicine and Bioethics*. 36 (5). 299–320.

Kristjánsson, K. (2015b) *Aristotelian Character Education*. Abingdon: Routledge.

Kristjánsson, K., Arthur, J., Moller, F. and Huo, Y. (2017) *Character and Virtues in Business and Finance*. Birmingham: Jubilee Centre for Character and Virtues.

Kristjánsson, K., Varghese, J., Arthur, J. and Moller, F. and Ferkany, M. (2017) *Virtuous Practice in Nursing*. Birmingham: Jubilee Centre for Character and Virtues.

Lievens, F. and Patterson, F. (2011) 'The validity and incremental validity of knowledge tests, low-fidelity simulations and high-fidelity simulations for predicting job performance in advanced-level high-stakes selection', *Journal of Applied Psychology*. 96 (5). 927–940.

Lipscomb, M. (2019) 'Neoliberalism and neoliberals: What are we talking about?' *Nursing Inquiry*. 27 (1). https://doi.org/10.1111/nin.12318.

McKie, A., Baguley, F., Guthrie, C., Jackons, C., Kirkpatrick, P., Laing, A., O'Brien, S., Taylor, R. and Wimpenny, P. (2012) 'Exploring clinical wisdom in nursing education', *Nursing Ethics*. 19 (2). 252–267.

Mercile, J. (2018) 'Neoliberalism and health care: The case of the Irish nursing home sector', *Critical Public Health*. 28 (5). 546–559.

Moore, G. (2015) 'Corporate character, corporate virtues', *Business Ethics: A European Review*. 24 (2). 99–114.

Nathaniel, A. (2006) 'Moral reckoning in nursing', *Western Journal of Nursing Research*. 28 (4). 419–438.

National Health Service England (2012) *Compassion in Practice: Nursing, Midwifery and Care Staff, Our Vision and Strategy*. London: NHS England.

Newham, R. A. (2015) 'Virtue ethics and nursing: On what grounds?' *Nursing Philosophy*. 16 (1). 40–50.

Nursing and Midwifery Council (2019) *Realising Professionalism: Standards for Education and Training*. London: NMC.

Nursing and Midwifery Council (2020) *The Code: Professional Standards of Practice and Behaviour for Nurses, Midwives and Nursing Associates*. London: NMC.

Oakley, J. and Cocking, D. (2001) *Virtue Ethics and Professional Roles*. Cambridge: Cambridge University Press.

Patterson, F. and Ashworth, V. (2011) 'Situational judgement tests: The future of medical selection?' http://careers.bmj.com/careers/advice/view-article.html?id=20005183; accessed 2 April 2021.

Pavlish, C., Brown-Saltzman, K., Jakel, P. and Fine, A. (2014) 'The nature of ethical conflicts and the meaning of moral community in oncology practice', *Oncology Nursing Forum*. 41 (2). 130–140.

Pellegrino, E. and Thomasma, D. (1993) *The Virtues in Medical Practice*. Oxford: Oxford University Press.

Peterson, A. and Arthur, J. (2020) *Ethics and the Good Teacher: Character in the Professional Domain*. Abingdon: Routledge.

Peterson, C. and Park, N. (2009) 'Classifying and Measuring Strengths of Character', in Lopez, S. J. and Snyder, C. R. (eds.) *Oxford Handbook of Positive Psychology*, 2nd edition, New York, NY: Oxford University Press, pp. 25–33.

Peterson, C. and Seligman, M. E. P. (2004) *Character Strengths and Virtues: A Handbook and Classification*. New York, NY: Oxford University Press.

Pitman, A. (2012) 'Professionalism and professionalization: Hostile ground for growing phronesis', in E. A. Kinsella and A. Pitman (eds.) *Phronesis as Professional Knowledge: Practical Wisdom in the Professions*. Rotterdam: Sense, pp. 131–146.

Poorchangizi, B., Farokhzadian, J., Abbaszadeh, A., Mirzaee, M. and Borhani, F. (2017) 'The importance of professional values from clinical nurses' perspective in hospitals of a medical university in Iran', *BMC Medical Ethics*. 18 (1). 1–7.

Repenshek, M. (2009) 'Moral distress: Inability to act or discomfort with moral subjectivity?' *Nursing Ethics*. 16 (6), 734–742.

Rhodes, R. (2020) *The Trusted Doctor: Medical Ethics and Professionalism*. Oxford: Oxford University Press.

Ritchie, J. and Spencer, L. (1994) 'Qualitative data analysis for applied policy research', in A. Bryman and R. G. Burgess (eds.) *Analysing Qualitative Data*. London: Routledge, pp. 173–194.

Royal Pharmaceutical Society (2011) 'Reducing workplace pressure through professional empowerment', www.rpharms.com/Portals/0/RPS%20document%20library/Open%20access/Support/64585_Reducing%20Workplace%20Pressure%20through%20professional%20empowerment%20-%20FINAL.PDF?ver=2017-05-16-133220-000; accessed 20 November 2020.

Russell, D. (2009) *Practical Intelligence and the Virtues*. Oxford: Oxford University Press.

Seijts, G., Crossan, M. and Carleton, E. (2017) 'Embedding leader character into HR practices and to achieve sustained excellence', *Organizational Dynamics*. 44 (1). 65–74.

Schwartz, B. (2009) 'Our loss of wisdom', *TED2009*. www.ted.com/talks/barry_schwartz_our_loss_of_wisdom? accessed 24 November 2019.

Schwartz, B. (2011) 'Using our practical wisdom', *TEDSalon New York*. www.ted.com/talks/barry_schwartz_using_our_practical_wisdom?language=en; accessed 24 November 2019.

Sellman, D. (2009) 'Practical wisdom in health and social care: Teaching for professional phronesis', *Learning in Health and Social Care*. 8 (2). 84–91.

Sellman, D. (2011) *What Makes a Good Nurse: Why the Virtues Are Important for Nurses*. London: Jessica Kingsley Publishers.

Sellman, D. (2012) 'Reclaiming competence for professional phronesis', in E. A. Kinsella and A. Pitman (eds.) *Phronesis as Professional Knowledge: Practical Wisdom in the Professions*. Rotterdam: Sense, pp. 115–130.

Thompson, A., Maile, A. and Hollowood, L. (2021) *Bringing Character to Life: Virtues in Nursing*. Birmingham: Jubilee Centre for Character and Virtues, University of Birmingham.

Titchen, A. (2000) 'Professional craft knowledge in patient-centred nursing and facilitation of its development', D. Phil., University of Oxford.

Tollefsen, A. S., Olsen, A. B. and Clancy, A. (2021) 'Nurses' experiences of ethical responsibility: A hermeneutic phenomenological design', *Nordic Journal of Nursing Research*. 41 (1). 34–41.

Tronto, J. C. (1994) *Moral Boundaries. A Political Argument for an Ethic of Care*. New York: Routledge.

Tschudin, V. (2010) 'Nursing ethics: The last decade', *Nursing Ethics*. 17 (1). 127–131.

Tuckett, A. G. (2000) 'Virtuous principles as an ethic for nursing', *Contemporary Nurse*. 9 (2). 106–114.

Van Hooft, S. (1999) 'Acting from the virtue of caring in nursing', *Nursing Ethics*. 6. 189–201.

Vanlaere, L. and Gastmans, C. (2007) 'Ethics in nursing education: Learning to reflect on care practices', *Nursing Ethics*. 14 (6). 758–766.

Varghese, J. and Kristjánsson, K. (2018) 'Experienced UK nurses and the missing U-curve of virtue-based reasoning', in D. Carr (ed.) *Cultivating Moral Character and Virtue in Professional Practice*. Abingdon: Routledge, pp. 151–165.

West, A. (2017) 'The ethics of professional accountants: An Aristotelian perspective', *Accounting, Auditing & Accountability Journal*. 30 (2). 328–351.

Worth, J. and Van Den Brande, J. (2019) 'Teacher labour market in England: Annual report 2019', www.nfer.ac.uk/media/3344/teacher_labour_market_in_england_2019.pdf; accessed 20 November 2020.

Wright, J., Warren, M. and Snow, N. (2021) *Understanding Virtue*: *Theory and Measurement*. Oxford: Oxford University Press.

Wu, L. T., Low, M. M., Tan, K. K., Lopez, V. and Liaw, S. Y. (2015) 'Why not nursing? A systematic review of factors influencing career choice among healthcare students', *International Nursing Review*. 62 (4). 547–562.

Index

Note: Page numbers in *italics* indicate a figure and page numbers in **bold** indicate a table on the corresponding page.

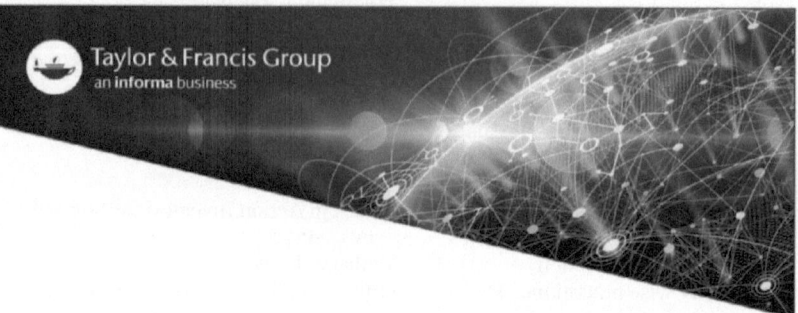
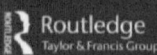
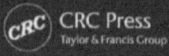